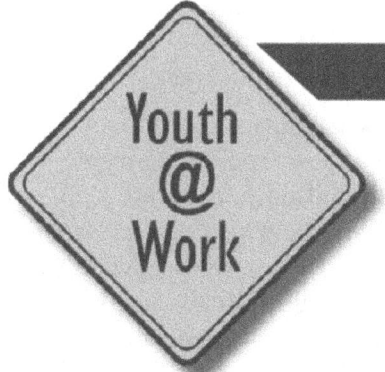

Youth @ Work

TALKING|SAFETY

TEACHING YOUNG WORKERS ABOUT JOB SAFETY AND HEALTH
NORTH CAROLINA EDITION

A joint publication of . . .

Centers for Disease Control and Prevention
National Institute for Occupational Safety and Health

Labor Occupational Health Program
University of California, Berkeley

Education Development Center, Inc.

2010

Preface/Introduction

NIOSH is pleased to present *Youth @ Work—Talking Safety*, a foundation curriculum in occupational safety and health. This curriculum is the culmination of many years' work by a consortium of partners dedicated to reducing occupational injuries and illnesses among youth. The initial curricula upon which *Youth @ Work—Talking Safety* is based included *WorkSafe!*, developed by the Labor Occupational Health Program (LOHP) at the University of California, Berkeley, and *Safe Work/Safe Workers*, developed by the Occupational Health Surveillance Program at the Massachusetts Department of Public Health and the Education Development Center, Inc. (EDC) in Newton, MA. Those products were produced under grants from NIOSH as well as the Occupational Safety and Health Administration, US Department of Labor; the Massachusetts Department of Industrial Accidents; the Maternal and Child Health Bureau, Health Resources and Services Administration; and Liberty Mutual Insurance Company.

The activities in the *Youth @ Work* curriculum were developed in consultation with numerous teachers and staff from general high schools, school to work, work experience, and vocational education programs, as well as the California WorkAbility program, which serves students with cognitive and learning disabilities. The activities have been extensively pilot tested and used by numerous high school teachers, job trainers, and work coordinators around the country to teach youth important basic occupational safety and health skills. In 2004, NIOSH made a commitment to integrate an occupational safety and health curriculum into US high schools. As part of this effort, the States' Career Clusters Initiative which operates under the auspices of the National Association of State Directors of Career Technical Education consortium (NASDCTEc) joined the partnership. The *Youth @ Work* curriculum was evaluated in sixteen schools across ten states during the 2004-2005 school year. This final version reflects the input from all of the teachers, administrators, students, and partners who participated in that evaluation.

Authors

Youth @ Work was based on materials originally authored by Diane Bush, Robin Dewey, and Betty Szudy of LOHP and Christine Miara of EDC. Additional contributors to *Youth @ Work* include Dr. Carol Stephenson, Dr. Andrea Okun, and Dr. Ted Fowler of NIOSH, and Dr. Frances Beauman from Illinois Office of Educational Services at Southern Illinois University.

Acknowledgements

This This curriculum was developed under the leadership of Dr. Paul Schulte, Director of the Education and Information Division at NIOSH. Funds were also provided by grant number H610-HT12 from the Occupational Safety and Health Administration (OSHA), US Department of Labor. Editors of this curriculum were Gene Darling (LOHP) and John Diether (NIOSH). Graphic and layout editor was Kate Oliver (LOHP), and illustrations provided by Mary Ann Zapalac (LOHP) and Pat Haskins (NIOSH). Technical reviewers included Dr. Letitia Davis (MA Department of Public Health), Mary Miller (WA Department of Labor and Industries), Elise Handelman (OSHA), and representatives of various professional and educational organizations such as the American Industrial Hygiene Association, The American Society of Safety Engineers, and the National Safety Council. Additional NIOSH contributors to the 2010 version include Rebecca Guerin (content editor) and Stephen Leonard (web designer I desktop publisher).

We would like to thank the many teachers, administrators, and students from the participating schools and states who evaluated the 2004-2005 pilot curriculum:

East Valley Institute of Technology, Mesa, AZ
Tampa Bay Technical High School, Tampa, FL
Mid Florida Tech, Orlando, FL
West Florida High School of Advanced Technology, Pensacola, FL
Professional/Technical Education Center (PTEC), Boise, ID
Herrin High School, Herrin, IL
Kankakee Valley High School, Wheatfield, IN
Millcreek Center, Olathe, KS
Landry High School, New Orleans, LA
Mandeville High School, Mandeville, LA
Walker High School, Walker, LA
Lewis & Clark Career Center, St. Charles, MO
Whitmer High School, Toledo, OH
Lenepe Technical School, Ford City, PA
State College Area School District & CTE Center, State College, PA

Disclaimers:

Mention of any company or product does not constitute endorsement by the National Institute for Occupational Safety and Health (NIOSH). In addition, citations to Web sites external to NIOSH do not constitute NIOSH endorsement of the sponsoring organizations or their programs or products. Furthermore, NIOSH is not responsible for the content of these Web sites.

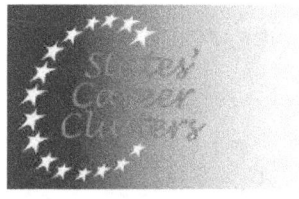

*Youth @ Work — **Talking Safety** is endorsed by the **States' Career Clusters Initiative** (2006). Endorsement does not carry with it any legal, fiscal, policy or other responsibility or liability by the endorser for this product. Endorsement means the product aligns to and supports the general spirit, intent and goals of the **States' Career Clusters Initiative**. Endorsement does not imply priority or preference of any product.* www.careerclusters.org

Readers are free to duplicate any and all parts of this publication; however, in accordance with standard publishing practices, NIOSH appreciates acknowledgement of any information reproduced.

For more information:

NIOSH   www.cdc.gov/niosh

Labor Occupational Health Program (LOHP)
University of California at Berkeley
2223 Fulton Street
Berkeley, CA 94720-5120
Phone: (510) 642-5507
Fax: (510) 643-5698
www.lohp.org
E-mail: lohp@socrates.berkeley.edu

Education Development Center, Inc. (EDC)
55 Chapel Street, Newton, Massachusetts 02458-1060
Phone: (617) 969-7100
Fax: (617) 969-5979
TTY: (617) 964-5448
 www.edc.org

Career Clusters www.careerclusters.org

National Association of State Directors of Career Technical Education Consortium (NASDCTEc)
www.careertech.org

Pub no 2007-136(NC)

Table of Contents

Overheads

Student Handouts

Appendices

A. Optional Student Handout: Hazards in Typical Teen Jobs

B. Certificate of Completion

Introduction

Why Teach Young Workers About Job Safety and Health?

Millions of teens in the United States work. Surveys indicate that 80% of teens have worked by the time they finish high school. While work provides numerous benefits for young people, it can also be dangerous. Every year, approximately 53,000 youth are injured on the job seriously enough to seek emergency room treatment. In fact, teens are injured at a higher rate than adult workers.

As new workers, adolescents are likely to be inexperienced and unfamiliar with many of the tasks required of them. Yet despite teen workers' high job injury rates, safety at work is usually one of the last things they worry about. Many of teens' most positive traits—energy, enthusiasm, and a need for increased challenge and responsibility—can result in their taking on tasks they are not prepared to do safely. They may also be reluctant to ask questions or make demands on their employers.

Health and safety education is an important component of injury prevention for working teens. While workplace-specific training is most critical, young people also need the opportunity to learn and practice general health and safety skills that they will carry with them from job to job. Teens should be able to recognize hazards in any workplace. They should understand how hazards can be controlled, what to do in an emergency, what rights they have on the job, and how to speak up effectively when problems arise at work.

School and community-based programs that place youth in jobs offer an important venue for teaching these skills. One national program that recognizes the importance of including these skills as part of the educational experience is the Career Cluster Initiative, developed by the U.S. Department of Education Office of Vocational and Adult Education (OVAE) and currently being implemented in a number of states. OVAE identified 16 career clusters that include the major job opportunities in today's workforce. Examples of clusters are finance, architecture and construction, and health science. (For a complete list of career clusters, see *www.careerclusters.org*.) Each cluster has a curriculum framework and a set of core knowledge and skills students should master, which includes workplace health and safety.

Youth @ Work: Talking Safety

This curriculum has been designed to teach core health and safety skills and knowledge, covering basic information relevant to any occupation.

The learning activities in this curriculum are intended to raise awareness among young people about occupational safety and health and provide them with the basic skills they need to become active participants in creating safe and healthy work environments.

The activities highlight hazards and prevention strategies from a wide variety of workplaces. The materials are very flexible. They may be used as a stand-alone curriculum or may be incorporated into other safety programs. Teachers who have used this curriculum indicated that the material was an excellent introduction to other safety instruction such as the OSHA 10-hour course or occupational specific safety instruction. They also said it could be used to enhance other safety programs. Educators can tailor the curriculum to students in a specific career cluster by selecting the workplace examples and scenarios provided which are most relevant to that career cluster.

This curriculum has been endorsed by the U.S. Department of Education's Career Cluster Initiative, Job Corps, and Skills USA.

Overview of the Curriculum

Youth @ Work: Talking Safety is designed to help teachers, as well as school and community-based job placement staff, give young people the basics of job health and safety in a fun and interesting way. The curriculum presents essential information and skills through a focus on six topic areas:

Lesson 1, *Young Worker Work Injuries*, assesses students' current knowledge of job safety and legal rights. It also introduces students to these issues and emphasizes the impact a job injury can have on a young person's life.

Lesson 2, *Finding Hazards*, develops an understanding of the common health and safety hazards that teens may face on the job.

Lesson 3, *Finding Ways To Make the Job Safer*, explains measures that can reduce or eliminate hazards on the job. It also shows students how to get more information about specific hazards they may face and on how to control them.

Lesson 4, *Emergencies at Work*, introduces students to the various types of emergencies that may occur in a workplace, and how the employer and workers should respond to them.

Lesson 5, *Know Your Rights*, focuses on the legal rights all workers have under health and safety laws, the special rights young workers have under child labor laws, and the government agencies and other resources that can help. Be sure to obtain the version of this curriculum that is specific to your state because some laws and agency names vary from state to state. Download from: *www.cdc.gov/NIOSH*.

Lesson 6, *Taking Action*, helps develop skills in speaking up effectively if a problem arises at work.

Lesson Plans, Overheads, and Student Handouts are provided for all six lessons. The 13-minute video presented in Lesson 1 is also included. The Appendix includes an optional handout which gives more information about hazards in typical teen jobs. A Certificate of Completion is also provided and may be photocopied.

Lessons may be presented together or over several class periods. Included in each lesson are:

- Learning Objectives (what the students will learn).

- A Lesson Plan chart with a short summary of the activities included, the time required for each activity, and the materials needed.

- A section titled Preparing To Teach This Lesson, with a list of steps to follow when you prepare—obtain equipment, prepare handouts, etc.

- Detailed Instructor's Notes with complete teaching instructions.

- Tips for a Shorter Lesson (suggestions for covering the material in less time).

Each lesson begins with an introductory discussion, followed by two or three participatory learning activities for teaching the concepts of that lesson. At least one of the learning activities in each lesson is very basic, with minimal or no reading required, and is designed to meet the needs of all students. Several of these activities have been developed for, and pilot tested with, students who have cognitive and learning disabilities.

As you prepare to teach this course, look through all the activities that make up each lesson. Select the activities that you feel will be most effective with your particular students. The curriculum is very flexible and gives you many alternatives from which to choose.

The time required for each activity within a lesson is shown in the Lesson Plan chart at the beginning of the lesson. This entire course can be taught in three to five hours, depending upon whether you teach one activity, or all activities, from each lesson. If you have less than three hours to devote to this topic, consult the section at the end of each lesson called "Tips for a Shorter Lesson."

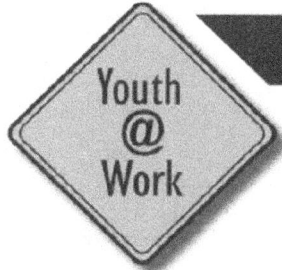
LESSON ONE
YOUNG WORKER INJURIES

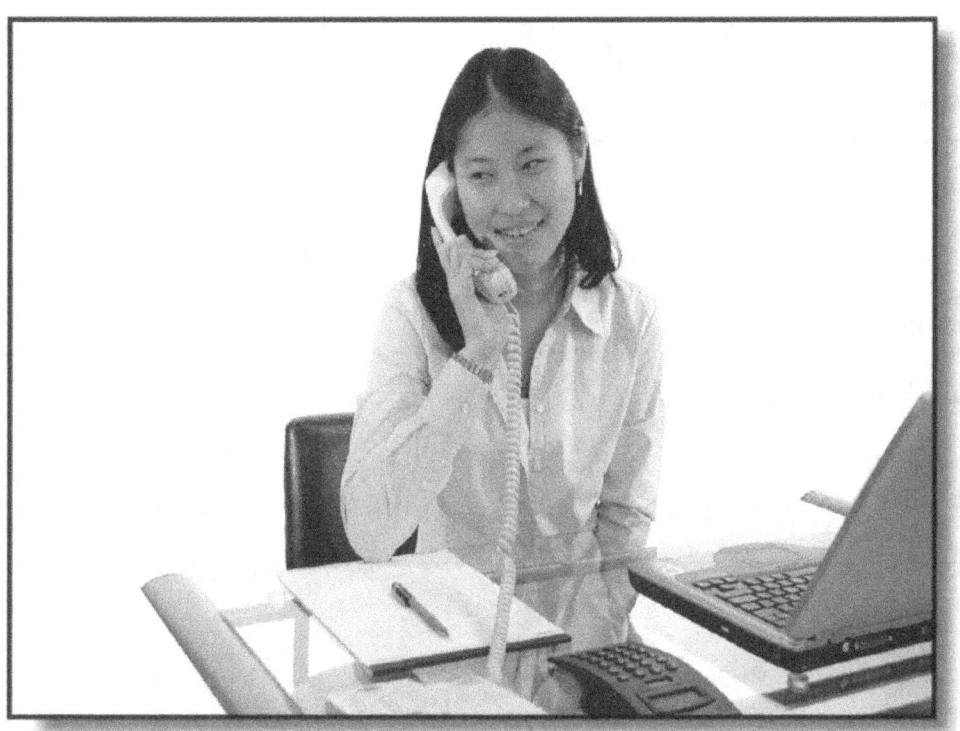

Learning Objectives

By the end of this lesson, students will be able to:

Determine how much they already know about job safety and their legal rights.

Describe the impact work injuries can have on a young person's life.

Identify the major messages in a video on teen job safety.

Define the word "hazard" and identify possible health and safety hazards in the workplaces shown in the video.

Lesson Plan One

	Activity	Time	Materials
A.	**Introduction: Young workers and safety.** Students participate in a "warm-up" discussion about what jobs they have had, and whether they have ever been injured at work.	15 minutes	• Flipchart & markers, or chalkboard & chalk. • Overheads #1–5.
B.	**Your safety IQ quiz.** Students work together in small groups on a quiz that tests their current safety knowledge. The whole class then reviews answers.	10 minutes	• Overhead #6. • Student Handout #1.
C.	**Video and discussion.** The instructor leads a class discussion about the issues raised in the video, *Teen Workers: Real Jobs, Real Risks.*	15 minutes	• Video, DVD Player, and TV.
D.	**Goals of this training.** Instructor explains the goals of this series of classes.	5 minutes	• Overhead #7.

Preparing To Teach This Lesson

Before you present Lesson One:

1. Obtain a flipchart and markers, or use a chalkboard and chalk.

2. Copy each Overhead used in this lesson (#1–7) onto a transparency to show with an overhead projector.

3. Photocopy Student Handout #1, *Your Safety IQ Quiz*, for each student.

4. Obtain a DVD Player and TV.

5. Preview the provided video *Teen Workers: Real Jobs, Real Risks*.

Detailed Instructor's Notes

A. Introduction: Young workers and safety.
(15 minutes)

1. Explain that this is a series of classes about staying safe at work. Many teens have jobs, and sometimes their work is dangerous. Students in these classes will learn about:

   - Some of the ways people (both youth and adults) can get hurt on the job.

   - What to do if you see something at work that could hurt you or make you sick.

   - What legal rights **all** workers have to make sure their jobs are safe.

   - What extra protections **young** workers have under child labor laws.

2. As a warm-up discussion, ask students:

> "How many of you have ever had a job?"

> "Where did you work?"

> "What did you do?"

> "Have you ever been hurt at work, or do you know someone who was?"

> "Have you ever been afraid about a task you've been asked to do at work?"

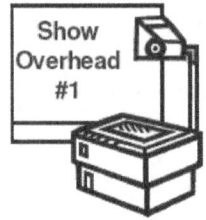

Let the class briefly discuss their answers. The questions are designed to get students thinking about safety issues in their own job experience.

3. To emphasize the impact work injuries can have on a young person's life, tell about an actual news story from your state or read the class at least one of the stories below. Or you can select stories from Lesson 3 (B), the $25,000 Safety Pyramid game (pages 28–33). All stories are based on injuries that actually occurred.

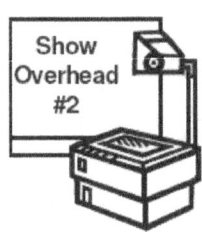

John worked at a fast food restaurant. The floor often got very greasy, and had to be washed a lot. As John walked across the wet floor, carrying a basket of french fries, he slipped. He tried to keep the fries from falling, so he couldn't break his fall with his hands. He fell on his tailbone and was seriously injured. He is now permanently disabled and has trouble walking.

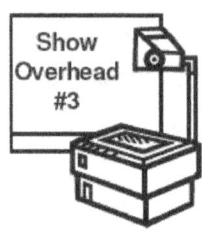

Antonio worked for a neighborhood builder. One day when he was carrying a 12-foot roof rafter along the top of an unfinished house, he backed into an unguarded chimney hole and plunged 28 feet to a concrete cellar floor below. He survived, but with three cracked vertebrae that forced him to spend the next three months locked in a "clamshell" brace from his neck to his hips.

Keisha did much of her homework on the computer and spent time each day e-mailing her friends. In addition, she worked three hours a day after school inputting data for a direct mail company. She was paid by "piece work" (by the amount of work, not the amount of time). She never took breaks. She began getting numbness in her fingers and waking up with a burning sensation in her wrist. Her doctor told her she has severe repetitive stress injury (RSI), in which prolonged typing in

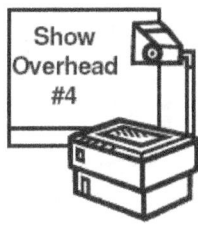

an awkward position damages muscles, tendons, and nerves. She now must wear braces on her wrists day and night and can't work on the computer for more than 15 minutes at a time. Her high school has arranged for someone to take notes in class for her, and when she goes to college she will have to use special software that allows her to dictate rather than type her papers.

Francisco was a 15-year-old boy who found work with a landscape company after moving to Maryland with his family. After only a week on the job he was assigned to help spread mulch at a large residence using a motorized grinding mulch blower. Somehow, he got up where the mulch mix is fed into the top of the machine, and fell into the grinding machinery of the mulch-spreading truck. A co-worker found his remains soon after.

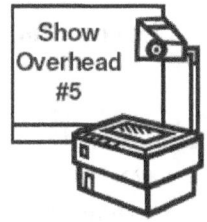

4. Ask students the questions below about each story you read.

   As people respond, write what they say on a flipchart page. (You don't need to discuss the answers now. Explain that students will learn more about these issues during the training.)

   "Why do you think this happened?"

   "What could have prevented this person from getting hurt?"

5. Show Overhead #5. Tell students that more teens tend to be injured in the industries where a lot of young people work. Since a little over 50% of teens work in retail, which includes fast food restaurants, most injuries occur in retail.

B. Your safety IQ quiz.
(10 minutes)

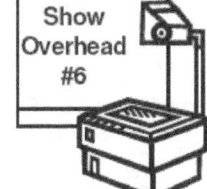

1. Explain that this quiz is designed to help students find out how much they already know about workplace health and safety and workers' rights. They will work together in small groups. They can guess at answers if they are not sure. Each group should choose someone to report the group's answers to the class later.

2. Give everyone a copy of Student Handout #1, *Your Safety IQ Quiz.*

3. Break the class into small groups of 4–6 students.

4. Circulate among the groups to see how they are doing.

5. After 5 minutes, bring the class back together.

6. Call on the first group's reporter. Have this student read the first question, give the group's answer, and explain it. Have the class discuss this answer.

7. Call on other groups in turn until all five questions have been answered. Make a check mark beside the correct answer on Overhead #6 after you answer each question.

8. Use the answer key below to help clarify the correct answers if needed. Explain that students will learn more about these topics during this training.

✔ Your Safety IQ—Questions and Discussion Points

1. **True or False? The law says your employer must give you training about health and safety hazards on your job.**

    True. You should get training before you start work. The training should cover how to do your job safely. Training about hazardous chemicals and other health and safety hazards at your job is required by OSHA (the Occupational Safety and Health Administration), the agency that enforces workplace health and safety laws.

2. **True or False? The law sets limits on how late you may work on school a night if you are under 16.**

    True. The federal law says if you are 14 or 15, you can only work until 7pm on a school night. Some **states** also have restrictions on how late you can work if you are 16 or 17. Child labor laws protect teens from working too late, too early, or too long.

3. **True or False? If you are 16 years old you are allowed to drive a car on public streets as part of your job.**

    False. Teens who are 16 may not drive a car or truck on public streets as part of their job. Federal law permits teens who are 17 to drive in very limited situations. Some states do not allow anyone under 18 to drive on the job. Child labor laws protect teens from doing dangerous work.

4. **True or False? If you're injured on the job, your employer must pay for your medical care.**

True. If you get hurt on the job, the law says your employer must provide workers' compensation benefits. These include medical care for your injury.

5. How many teens get injured on the job in the U.S.?

☐ One per day   ☐ One per hour   ☐ One every 10 minutes

One every 10 minutes. Overall, 53,000 teens are hurt each year badly enough to go to a hospital emergency room. Only one-third of work-related injuries are seen in emergency rooms, so it is likely that more than 150,000 teens suffer work-related injuries each year. About 48 U.S. teens (17 and under) die each year from job injuries. Teens are often injured on the job due to unsafe equipment or stressful conditions. They also may not receive enough safety training and supervision.

9. Tell students that one of the reasons both young and older workers get injured at work is because there are **hazards** (dangers) on the job. Write the definition of the word "hazard" on the flipchart or chalkboard:

   A hazard is anything at work that can hurt you, either physically or mentally.

   Explain that the class will talk more about hazards in the workplace after they watch a video about working teens and safety.

C. Video and discussion.
(15 minutes)

1. Explain that the class will now watch a 13-minute video called *Teen Workers: Real Jobs, Real Risks.* The video introduces some of the topics that will be covered in this series of classes.

   Ask students to keep in mind these questions while they watch the tape:

   "What are the main messages of the video? What are the teens in the video trying to tell you?"

   "What are some health or safety hazards you see on the jobs shown in the video?"

2. Show the video.

---

3. After the video, hold a class discussion. First, ask students to list what they believe were the main messages. What did the teens in the video want them to know? Let volunteers answer. Possible messages include:

- There are hazards on most jobs.

- Teens do get injured at work.

- Teens have rights on the job.

- Teens should speak up and ask questions if they are concerned about something at work.

- There are ways to reduce hazards on the job. Injuries can be prevented.

- Employers have a responsibility to make the workplace safe for workers.

4. Next, ask:

❝What job hazards did you notice in the video?❞

Possible answers include:

- Dangerous / unguarded machinery.

- Meat slicer.

- Lifting boxes and other containers.

- Hot liquids / fryers.

- Congested work areas.

- Time pressures / fast-paced work environment.

- Working around money.

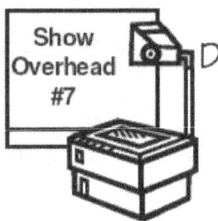
Show Overhead #7

D. Goals of this training.
(5 minutes)

1. Explain that this series of lessons will help students avoid becoming part of the injury statistics. They will learn about workplace health and safety, as well as teen workers' rights on the job.

2. Explain that during the training, students will participate in several different activities: drawing maps that show hazards in the workplace, role plays, and games. By the end they will know more about:

- Identifying and reducing hazards on the job

- Laws that protect teens from working too late or too long

- Laws that protect teens from doing dangerous work

- How to solve health and safety problems at work

- What agencies enforce health and safety laws and child labor laws

- What to do in different kinds of emergencies.

Tips for a Shorter Lesson

A shorter version of Lesson One can be presented in 20–30 minutes by beginning with the Introduction and then presenting either the quiz or the video.

1. **Introduction: Young workers and safety** (15 minutes). Students participate in a warm-up discussion about teens and safety.

2. **Give quiz** (5–10 minutes). Ask the class as a whole to do the quiz (instead of small groups). Show the class Overhead #6 and have them brainstorm answers.

3. **Video and discussion** (15 minutes). The class watches *Teen Workers: Real Jobs, Real Risks* and discusses the video.

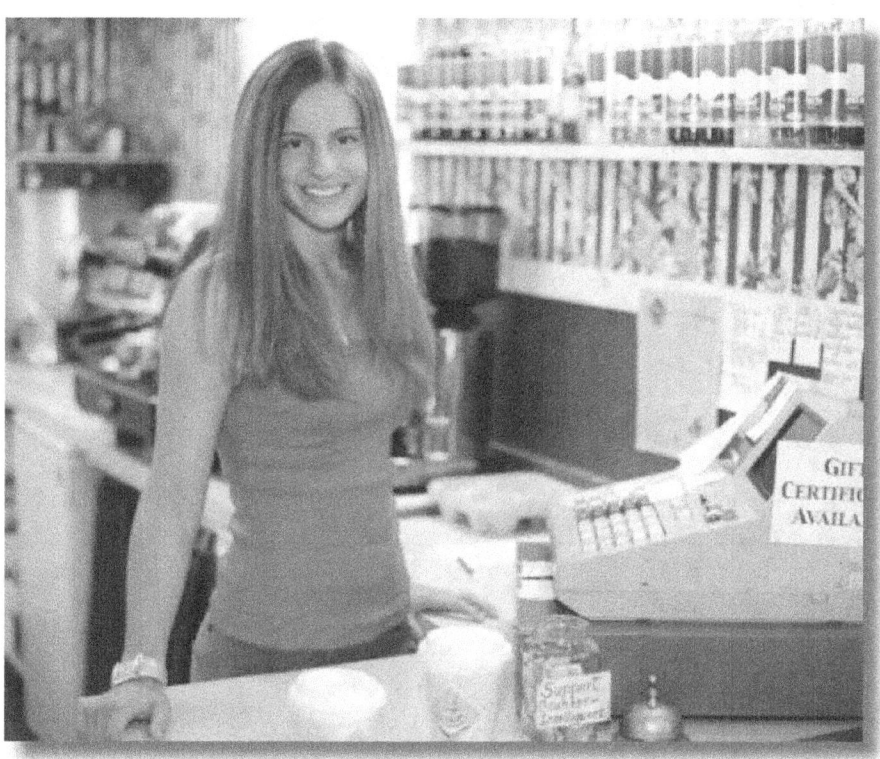

Learning Objectives

By the end of this lesson, students will be able to:

Identify a variety of health and safety hazards found at typical worksites that employ young people.

Locate various types of hazards in an actual workplace.

Identify the major messages in a video on teen job safety.

Explain how to get information about chemical hazards.

Lesson Plan Two

	Activity	Time	Materials
A.	**Introduction: What is a job hazard?** The class "brainstorms" to develop a list of possible workplace health and safety hazards.	10 minutes	• Flipchart & markers, or chalkboard & chalk. • Overhead #8.
B.	**Find the hazards in the picture.** Students work in pairs. They look at pictures of typical teen workplaces and try to identify health and safety hazards. Then students report back on the hazards they found.	20 minutes	• Overheads #9–12. • Student Handouts #2–5. • One colored marker per pair of students. • Erasable marker for transparencies.
C.	**Hazard mapping.** In small groups, students draw maps showing the location and types of hazards in typical workplaces. Then groups take turns explaining their maps.	30 minutes	• Overhead #13. • Flipchart paper and colored markers for groups.
D.	**Hunting for hazards.** Pairs of students walk through work areas at the school or at a nearby workplace. They search for health and safety hazards and record their findings.	30 minutes	• Student Handout #6. • Pens or pencils.
E.	**Review.** Instructor summarizes key points of this lesson.	5 minutes	• Overhead #14.

Preparing To Teach This Lesson

Before you present Lesson Two:

1. Decide which activities you will use to teach this lesson. We recommend you begin with the *Introduction* (A). Then use **either** *Find the hazards in the picture* (B) **or** *Hazard mapping* (C), depending on the level of your students. Teachers using this curriculum have found that, for some students, the *Hazard mapping* activity is too abstract. *Hunting for hazards* (D) can be used to reinforce either (B) or (C) as needed. If you have extra time, you can use all the activities.

2. Obtain a flipchart and markers, or use a chalkboard and chalk.

3. For the *Introduction*, copy Overhead #8 onto a transparency to show with an overhead projector.

4. For the *Find the hazards* activity, photocopy Student Handouts #2–5 (*Fast Food, Grocery Store, Office,* and *Gas Station*) so each pair of students will have one set. Also copy Overheads #9–12 onto transparencies. Obtain enough colored markers or pens so each pair of students will have one to mark their handouts. Also obtain an erasable marker to use with the transparencies.

5. For the *Hazard mapping* activity, obtain flipchart paper and a set of five colored markers (black, red, green, blue, orange) for each small group. Copy Overhead #13 onto a transparency.

6. For the *Hunting for hazards* activity, photocopy Student Handout #6, so each pair of students will have one copy. Arrange access to work areas.

7. Copy Overhead #14 onto a transparency for use in summarizing the main points of this lesson at the end of the class.

Detailed Instructor's Notes

A. Introduction: What is a job hazard?
(10 minutes)

1. Remind the class that a job hazard is anything at work that can hurt you, either physically or mentally.

   Explain that some job hazards are very obvious, but others are not. In order to be better prepared to be safe on the job, it is necessary to be able to identify different types of hazards.

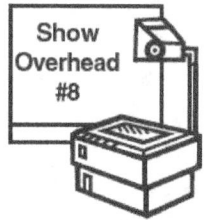

Show Overhead #8

Tell the class that hazards can be divided into four categories. Write the categories across the top of a piece of flipchart paper and show Overhead #8.

Safety hazards can cause immediate accidents and injuries. Examples: hot surfaces or slippery floors.

Chemical hazards are gases, vapors, liquids, or dusts that can harm your body. Examples: cleaning products or pesticides.

Biological hazards are living things that can cause diseases such as flu, AIDS, Hepatitis, Lyme Disease, and TB. Examples: bacteria, viruses, or insects. In the workplace, you can be exposed to biological hazards through contact with used needles, sick children, animals, etc.

Other health hazards are harmful things, not in the other categories, that can injure you or make you sick. These hazards are sometimes less obvious because they may not cause health problems right away. Examples: noise or repetitive movements.

2. Ask students to think about places they have worked, or workplaces with which they are familiar (restaurants, stores, theaters, offices, etc.).

Have students call out possible job hazards and say whether each one is a safety hazard, chemical hazard, biological hazard, or other health hazard. List each hazard in the matching column on the flipchart paper. Alternatively, have the class generate one list of hazards and then work in small groups to categorize them.

Note: Students may confuse the **effects** of hazards with the hazards themselves. They may mention "cuts" instead of knives, which cause the cuts. The **cause** is the hazard and should be listed on the chart. If people give effects rather than causes, ask them what **causes** the problem they mention. This will help later when students discuss how to eliminate hazards.

Your completed chart may be similar to this sample:

SAFETY HAZARDS	CHEMICAL HAZARDS	BIOLOGICAL HAZARDS	OTHER HEALTH HAZARDS
• hot surfaces • slippery floors • unsafe ladders • machines without guards • sharp knives • hot grease • unsafe electric circuits • lack of fire exits • motor vehicles • cluttered work areas • falling objects • violence	• cleaning products • pesticides • solvents • acids • asbestos • lead • ozone (from copiers) • wood dust • mercury • poor air quality • gasoline	• viruses • bacteria • molds • animals • birds • insects • poison ivy • poison oak • used needles	• noise • vibration • radiation • heat or cold • repetitive movements • awkward posture • heavy lifting • fast pace of work • harassment • stress • areas too dark or too bright

3. Add information about chemicals. Ask the class the following questions to prompt discussion:

❝How can chemicals get inside your body?❞

Answer: When you breathe them in, swallow them, or get them on your skin.

❝How can chemicals harm you?❞

Answer: Chemicals can cause many different kinds of symptoms, such as dizziness and breathing problems, and health effects like burns and more serious diseases like cancer, or failure of a vital organ such as the liver.

Some chemicals may cause both symptoms right away and other health problems that show up later in life. This is especially likely if you use certain chemicals for a long time.

❝What are some ways to find out how a chemical product might harm you and how to protect yourself from it?❞

Answer: When you use a product that contains chemicals (like a cleaning solution or a pesticide), it's important to know what kinds of health effects the chemical can cause, and how to protect yourself. If you already have asthma or some other health problem, this information can be especially important.

The Occupational Safety and Health Administration (OSHA) is the federal government agency that enforces worker health and safety laws. Some states also have state OSHA programs.

OSHA says that workers have a right to get information about the chemicals used in their workplace. Employers must train workers in how to use those chemicals safely, and teach them what to do if there is a chemical spill or other chemical emergency.

To find out more about the chemicals in a product, you can:

- Check the label

- Ask your supervisor

- Get training

- Call a resource agency or check their website

- Look at the Material Safety Data Sheet (MSDS) for the product.

OSHA requires employers to let their workers see and copy Material Safety Data Sheets (MSDSs) for every chemical used or stored at the workplace. MSDSs are information sheets that manufacturers must send to companies along with their chemical products. They tell you what is in the product, how it can harm you, and how to protect yourself.

The Environmental Protection Agency (EPA) also regulates the use of chemicals. They enforce the laws that protect our air, water, and soil from contamination.

B. Find the hazards in the picture.
(20 minutes)

1. Explain that each student will work with a partner on this activity. Divide the class into pairs.

2. Distribute materials. Pass out sets of "Find the Hazards" handouts (Student Handouts #2–5). Each pair of students should receive one set (all four handouts) to work on. Also give each pair a colored marker (such as a highlighter or pen).

3. Explain the activity. Each pair of students should look at the four workplaces shown in the handouts. In each workplace, they should try to find as many hazards as they can (either safety or health hazards). Using the colored marker, they should circle the hazards they find.

   Tell students they will have about 10 minutes to find all the hazards in the four pictures. Tell them they also should think about how each hazard could harm them if they were working in this workplace. They will be asked about this later.

4. After about 10 minutes, bring the class back together.

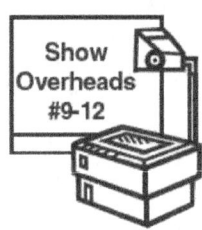

5. Overheads #9–12 have the same pictures that students looked at on their handouts. Show these one at a time. Have student volunteers circle on the overhead transparency the hazards they identified in each picture. Students may use an erasable marker directly on the transparency.

   After each Overhead is presented and marked, ask the whole class if they can think of additional hazards that the volunteers didn't find. Or are there hazards that could be present in that workplace, but are not shown in the picture? As students answer, mark these additional hazards on the transparency. If the class misses any hazards, point them out.

Show Overheads #9-12

Below is a list of hazards that are present in each illustrated workplace.

Fast Food

- Hot grill
- Fire
- Cooking grease
- Heavy lifting
- Cleaning chemicals
- Stress

- Steam
- Hot oven
- Knives
- Slippery floor
- Pressure to work fast

Grocery Store

- Heavy lifting
- Meat slicer
- Repetitive motion
- Standing a lot

- Box cutter
- Cleaning chemicals
- Bending or reaching
- Stress

Office

- Repetitive use of the keyboard
- Awkward posture
- Stress

- Cluttered workplace
- Copier and other chemicals

Gas Station

- Gasoline
- Heat or cold
- Stress

- Other chemicals
- Tools and equipment
- Violence

C. Hazard mapping.
(30 minutes)

1. Explain that students will work in small groups. Each group will choose or be assigned a type of workplace, and will draw a simple floor plan showing a typical workplace of that type. They will mark the location and type of hazards that may be found in that workplace. You and your students can choose workplaces where young workers often work, such as fast food restaurants, grocery stores, movie theaters, and offices. Appendix A contains a list of possible hazards in each of these four workplaces, for your information. Or you can select workplaces specifically relevant to your program or the experiences of your students.

2. Groups should draw their floor plans on flipchart paper, using a black marker. The floor plan should show rooms, work areas, furniture, equipment, work processes, doors, and windows. Explain that the floor plan can be very simple.

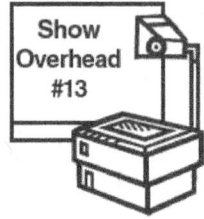

Show Overhead #13

3. Next, each group should mark the location of various hazards on their floor plans. Using the following color code can help reinforce the different categories of hazards. It's not necessary to color code the categories if it feels too complicated.

   Red to show safety hazards

   Green to show chemical hazards

   Orange to show biological hazards

   Blue to show other health hazards.

   Overhead #13 is a sample of a finished map.

4. (*Optional*) If you wish, also ask the groups to indicate how dangerous each hazard is. They can highlight hazards they consider especially serious or severe by coloring them more prominently.

5. Ask that each group choose someone to present their map to the entire class later. They should prepare to explain to the class what they believe are the major hazards in this workplace.

6. Divide the class into groups, with 3 or 4 students each. Assign or have them select the type of workplace they will draw. Give each group a large sheet of flipchart paper and five colored markers (black, red, green, orange, blue).

7. Answer any questions, and let the groups begin work. Circulate among the groups. Ask questions, make suggestions as appropriate. Challenge the students to think beyond obvious hazards. After about 15 minutes, bring the class back together.

8. Have the person selected by each group present and explain its map. The explanation should include a list of the major hazards in this type of workplace.

9. As each group presents its map, list any hazards people mention that were not previously listed on the chart created during the *Introduction*.

D. Hunting for hazards.
(30 minutes)

Note: Before beginning this activity, contact the appropriate staff around the school to ensure their support and cooperation.

1. Explain that each student will work with a partner on this activity. Divide the class into pairs.

2. Explain the activity. Tell students they will now look for health and safety hazards in a real workplace. If allowed by your school, pairs of students will walk to certain areas of the school and try to find hazards there. They will visit (for example) the school kitchen, the school office, and one other area of the school chosen by the instructor, such as a vocational shop.

   If the school does not have these facilities, the instructor should select other work areas in the school, or make arrangements to visit nearby workplaces.

3. Distribute materials. Give each pair of students a copy of the *Hunting for Hazards* form (Student Handout #6). Make sure each pair has a pen or pencil.

4. Pairs of students will now walk through the three selected areas of the school or other workplace, looking for health and safety hazards. Tell them to list the hazards they find in the correct section on Student Handout #6. For each hazard they identify, they should also write down how the hazard might harm someone working there.

5. Allow about 20 minutes for students to walk through all three work areas. When they have finished, bring the class back together to report what they found.

Notes to the instructor about this activity:

◆ This activity also can be done without using the form (Student Handout #6). Walk through the chosen work areas with students and ask them to point out hazards they see. Discuss as a group how each hazard they identify might harm someone.

◆ Consider conducting similar "walk-through inspections" of the workplaces where students will actually be working, to prepare them for their jobs.

◆ Consider reporting students' "findings" back to the teacher and/or administrator.

E. Review.

(5 minutes)

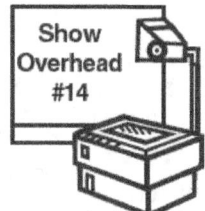

1. Review the key points covered in this lesson.

    •   Every job has health and safety hazards.

    •   You should always be aware of these hazards.

    •   You can find out about chemicals used at work by checking labels, reading Material Safety Data Sheets, and getting training. Your employer must provide training on how to work safely around chemicals.

Tips for a Shorter Lesson

A shorter version of Lesson Two can be presented in 20 minutes by brainstorming a list of hazards and then using a modified version of either the *Find the hazards in the picture* activity or the *Hazard mapping* activity.

1. **Brainstorm** (10 minutes). Explain what a job hazard is, and have the class quickly brainstorm a list of hazards in workplaces with which they are familiar. Prompt them to include chemical hazards and other less obvious hazards.

2. **Find the hazards in the picture** (10 minutes). Show Overheads #9–12 one at a time to the class. Have students call out the hazards they see and circle them on the transparency.

3. **Hazard mapping** (10 minutes). Using a black marker, draw a floorplan of a familiar workplace on flipchart paper in front of the class. (You may also ask a volunteer to do this.) Have the class supply important details. Have them suggest where to mark hazards on the map, and add them (in red).

LESSON THREE
MAKING THE JOB SAFER

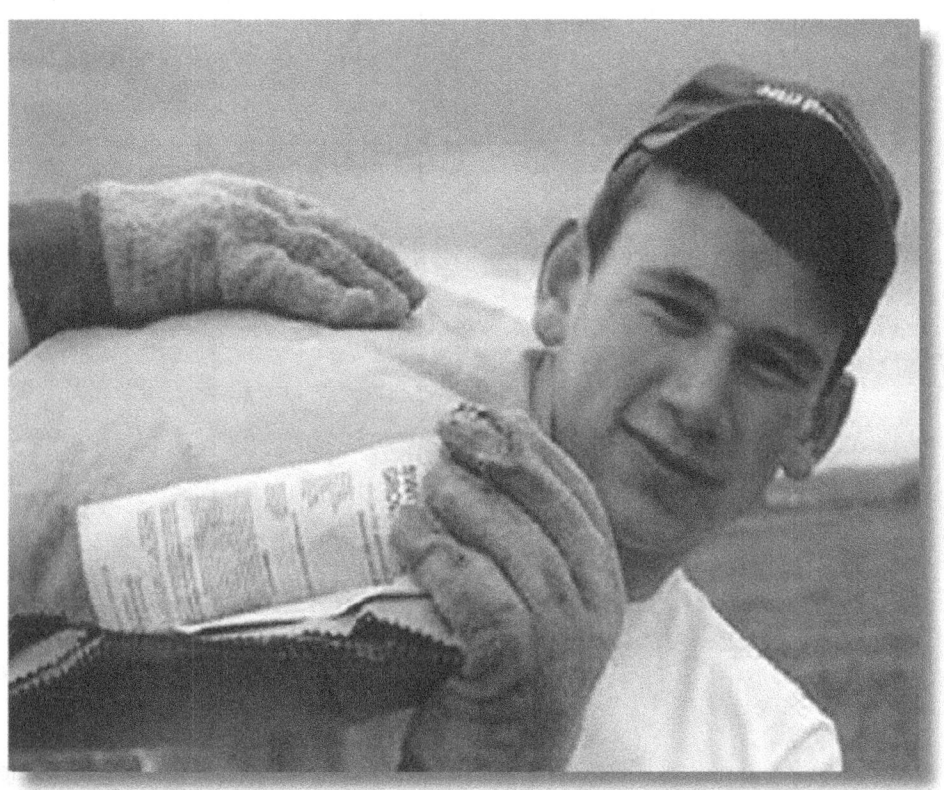

Learning Objectives

By the end of this lesson, students will be able to:

Describe the three main ways to reduce or eliminate hazards at work.

Explain which methods are most effective in controlling hazards.

Identify and describe at least three different sources of information on specific hazards, their health effects, and methods for controlling them.

Demonstrate the ability to find information to help address a specific hazard.

Lesson Plan Three

	Activity	Time	Materials
A.	**Introduction: Controlling hazards.** The class discusses the best ways to reduce or eliminate hazards on the job.	10 minutes	• Flipchart & markers, or chalkboard & chalk. • Overhead #15.
B.	**$25,000 Safety Pyramid game.** Teams of students play a game where they consider various work scenarios and come up with ideas for controlling the hazards shown. They organize their solutions into categories.	30 minutes	• Overheads #16–24. • Game board, score sheet, masking tape, and Post-its. • Watch or timer. • Pens or pencils. • Prizes. • Appendix A (optional).
C.	**Health and safety info search.** Students work in teams to research a specific health and safety problem, using the internet, phone, or other resources.	75 minutes	• Student Handout #7. • Internet or telephone access for students.
D.	**Review.** Instructor summarizes key points of this lesson.	5 minutes	• Overhead #25.

Preparing To Teach This Lesson

Before you present Lesson Three:

1. Obtain a flipchart and markers, or use a chalkboard and chalk.

2. Copy each Overhead used in this lesson (#15–25) onto a transparency to show with an overhead projector.

3. For the *$25,000 Safety Pyramid game* (B), draw a game board in advance on flipchart paper and tape it to the wall as described in section B. Also obtain pads of Post-it notes (a different color for each team), a watch or timer, and prizes (such as candy).

4. For the *Health and safety info search* activity (C), photocopy all pages of Student Handout #7 for each student. Also arrange for the class to have access to a computer with internet connection, a telephone, or both.

Detailed Instructor's Notes

A. Introduction: Controlling hazards.
(10 minutes)

1. On a piece of flipchart paper, create a table with two columns. Head the left column **Hazards** and the right column **Possible Solutions**.

2. Pick one job hazard from the list that the class made during Lesson Two. Write it in the **Hazards** column of the table. (For example, you might write "slippery floors.") Ask the class:

   ❝How can this workplace hazard be reduced or eliminated?❞

3. As students suggest answers, write them in the **Possible Solutions** column next to the hazard. Possible solutions for slippery floors might include:

   - Put out "Caution" signs.

   - Clean up spills quickly.

   - Install slip-resistant flooring.

   - Use floor mats.

   - Wear slip-resistant shoes.

   - Install grease guards on equipment to keep grease off the floor.

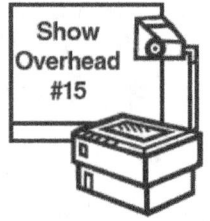

4. Explain to the class that there are often several ways to control a hazard, but some are better than others. Hold a class discussion of the three main control methods: remove the hazard, improve work policies and procedures, and use protective clothing and equipment.

Use Overhead #15 and the sections below to help explain these methods. After you discuss a method, apply it to the list you created on the flipchart, as indicated.

1. Remove the Hazard

The best control measures remove the hazard from the workplace altogether, or keep it isolated (away from workers) so it can't hurt anyone. This way, the workplace itself is safer, and all the responsibility for safety doesn't fall on individual workers.

Here are some examples:

- Use safer chemicals, and get rid of hazardous ones

- Store chemicals in locked cabinets away from work areas

- Use machines instead of doing jobs by hand

- Have guards around hot surfaces.

Ask the class:

❝Which of the solutions on the flipchart really get rid of the hazard of slippery floors?❞

Students should answer that slip-resistant flooring, floor mats, and grease guards are the items on the list that really remove the hazard. On the flipchart, put a "1" next to these solutions.

2. Improve Work Policies and Procedures

If you can't completely eliminate a hazard or keep it away from workers, good safety policies can reduce your exposure to hazards.

Here are some examples:

- Safety training on how to work around hazards

- Regular breaks to avoid fatigue

- Assigning enough people to do the job safely (lifting, etc.).

Ask the class:

❝Which of the solutions for slippery floors on the flipchart involve work policies and procedures?❞

Students should answer that putting out "Caution" signs and cleaning up spills quickly are in this category. On the flipchart, put a "2" next to these solutions.

3. Use Protective Clothing and Equipment

Personal protective equipment (often called "PPE") is the **least** effective way to control hazards. However, you should use it if it's all you have.

Here are some examples:

- Gloves, steel-toed shoes, hard hats

- Respirators, safety glasses, hearing protectors

- Lab coats or smocks.

Ask the class:

❝Why should PPE be considered the solution of last resort?❞

Answers may include:

- It doesn't get rid of or minimize the hazard itself.

- Workers may not want to wear it because it can be uncomfortable, hot, and may make it hard to communicate or do work.

- It has to fit properly and be used consistently at the right time to work.

- It has to be right for the particular hazard, such as the right respirator cartridge or glove for the chemical being used.

Ask the class:

❝Which of the solutions for slippery floors on the flipchart involve protective clothing and equipment?❞

Students should answer that wearing slip-resistant shoes is in this category. On the flipchart, put a "3" next to this solution.

When you have finished marking the three categories on the flipchart, your completed table may look like this:

HAZARD	POSSIBLE SOLUTIONS
Slippery floors	• Put out "Caution" signs. (2)
	• Clean up spills quickly. (2)
	• Install slip-resistant flooring. (1)
	• Use floor mats. (1)
	• Wear slip-resistant shoes. (3)
	• Install grease guards on equipment. (1)

Tell students that they will learn more about these control methods during the next activity. They will play a game called the $25,000 Safety Pyramid.

B. $25,000 Safety Pyramid game.
(30 minutes)

Instructor's Note. If you wish, you can present this material as a class discussion instead of a game. Show Overheads #16–24 to the class. For each Overhead, ask students for their ideas about possible ways to prevent the injuries described.

Prior to teaching this activity, review the stories (see pages 29–33 and Overheads #16–24) and select those stories most relevant to your students.

1. If you are presenting the material as a game, draw a game board like the one below on flipchart paper, and tape it to the wall.

$25,000 Safety Pyramid Game

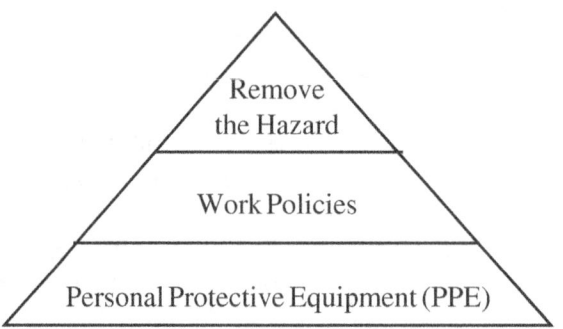

Remove the Hazard

Work Policies

Personal Protective Equipment (PPE)

2. Explain that in each round of the game, you will read aloud a true story about a youth who got injured at work.

   Students will work in teams. Teams should think of themselves as safety committees, responsible for finding ways to control the hazard that caused the injury described. Teams will be given a pad of Post-it notes on which to write their solutions.

   Notice that the pyramid divides solutions into three categories:

   - Remove the Hazard (often called engineering controls)

   - Work Policies (often called administrative controls)

   - Personal Protective Equipment (PPE).

   Explain that this is a fast-paced game and time counts. After you read each story, the teams will have one minute to come up with solutions and post them on the game board.

   One team member should be chosen as the "writer" for the team. Each solution the team comes up with should be written on a separate Post-it note. Another team member should be chosen as a "runner" who will post the team's notes in the correct categories on the game board.

   Tell the class that you will decide whether each solution is a good one. To be valid, it must:

   - Relate to the story

   - Be realistic

   - Be specific about the solution (for example, not just PPE, but *what kind* of PPE).

   Remember that some solutions may fall in more than one category. The same solution written on two Post-its placed in two categories should count once. Tell the class that in some cases there may be no good solutions in some of the categories. Explain that if teams put a good solution in the wrong category, you will move that Post-it to the proper category and give them the points.

   Explain that, after each round, you will tally the points. Each valid solution in the *Remove the Hazard* category is worth $2,000. Each valid solution in the *Work Policies* category is worth $1,000 and in the *PPE* category is worth $500 because these are usually less protective solutions, or solutions more prone to failure.

3. Select teams of 3-5 participants each. Ask each team to come up with a team name. Record team names on the chalkboard or on a sheet of flipchart paper, where you will keep track of the points.

   Pass out Post-it note pads, with a different color for each team.

4. Using Overhead #16, conduct a practice round. For this round, teams shouldn't bother writing down solutions, but should just call out their answers. Add any solutions the class misses.

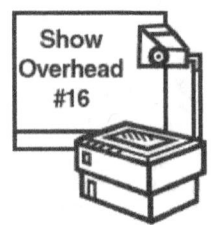

Practice Round: Jamie's Story

   Read the story aloud:

   Jamie is a 17-year-old dishwasher in a hospital kitchen. To clean cooking pans, she soaks them in a powerful chemical solution. She uses gloves to protect her hands and arms. One day, as Jamie was lifting three large pans out of the sink at once, they slipped out of her hands and back into the sink. The cleaning solution splashed all over the side of her face and got into her right eye. She was blinded in that eye for two weeks.

   Ask the class:

   > **"**What solutions can you think of that might prevent this injury from happening again?**"**

   > Suggested answers include:

   > **Remove the Hazard.** Substitute a safer cleaning product. Use disposable pans. Use a dishwashing machine.

   > **Work Policies.** Have workers clean one pan at a time. Give them training about how to protect themselves from chemicals.

   > **Personal Protective Equipment.** Goggles.

5. Begin the game. Play as many rounds as it takes for a team to reach $25,000. When a team wins, award prizes.

   At the end of each round, review the solutions teams have posted and total the points for valid answers. You can identify a team's solutions by the color of its Post-it notes. Add any solutions the teams missed.

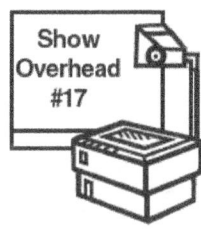

Round 1: Billy's Story

Read the story aloud:

Billy is a 16-year-old who works in a fast food restaurant. One day Billy slipped on the greasy floor. To catch his fall, he tried to grab a bar near the grill. He missed it and his hand touched the hot grill instead. He suffered second degree burns on the palm of his hand.

Ask the teams:

> **"**What solutions can you think of that might prevent this injury from happening again?**"**

> Give the teams one minute to write down their solutions and put them on the board. Then compare them to the suggested answers below.

> **Remove the Hazard.** Design the grill so the bar is not so close to the grill. Cover the floor with a non-skid mat. Install non-skid flooring. Put a shield on the grill when not in use to prevent people from accidentally touching it. Put a cover on the french-fry basket so grease won't splatter out.

> **Work Policies.** Have workers immediately clean up spilled grease. Design the traffic flow so workers don't walk past the grill.

> **Personal Protective Equipment.** Non-skid shoes. Gloves.

Round 2: Stephen's Story

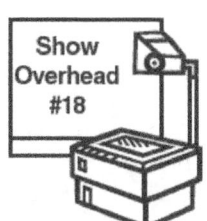

Read the story aloud:

Stephen is a 17-year-old who works in a grocery store. One day while unloading a heavy box from a truck onto a wooden pallet, he slipped and fell. He felt a sharp pain in his lower back. He was embarrassed, so he got up and tried to keep working. It kept bothering him, so he finally went to the doctor. He had to stay out of work for a week to recover. His back still hurts sometimes.

Ask the teams:

> **"**What solutions can you think of that might prevent this injury from happening again?**"**

> Have the teams post their solutions and compare them to the suggested answers below.

Remove the Hazard. Use a mechanical lifting device. Pack boxes with less weight. Unload trucks in a sheltered area so workers aren't exposed to weather, wind, or wet surfaces.

Work Policies. Assign two people to do the job. Train workers how to lift properly. Enforce a policy that teens never lift over 30 pounds at a time, as recommended by the National Institute for Occupational Safety and Health (NIOSH).

Personal Protective Equipment. Wear non-slip shoes. (Note: A recent NIOSH study found that back belts do not help. For more information see *www.cdc.gov/niosh/belting.html*.)

Then ask the class:

❝What is the proper way to lift heavy objects?❞

Demonstrate the following. Tell the class that the rules for safe lifting are:

1. Don't pick up objects over 30 pounds by yourself.

2. Keep the load close to your body.

3. Lift with your legs. Bend your knees and crouch down, keep your back straight, and then lift as you start to stand up.

4. Don't twist at your waist. Move your feet instead.

Round 3: Terry's Story

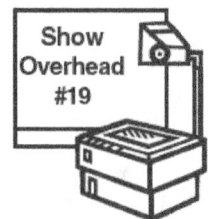

Show Overhead #19

Read the story aloud:

Terry is a 16-year-old who works in the deli department at a grocery store. Her supervisor asked her to clean the meat slicer, although she had never done this before and never been trained to do it. She thought the meat slicer was turned off before she began cleaning it. Just as she started to clean the blades, the machine started up. The blade cut a finger on Terry's left hand all the way to the bone.

Ask the teams:

❝What solutions can you think of that might prevent this injury from happening again?❞

Have the teams post their solutions and compare them to the suggested answers below.

Remove the Hazard. There should be a guard on the machine to protect fingers from the blade. There should be an automatic shut-off on the machine.

Work Policies. There should be a rule that the machine must be unplugged before cleaning. No one under 18 should be using or cleaning this machine because it is against the child labor laws.

Personal Protective Equipment. Cut-resistant gloves.

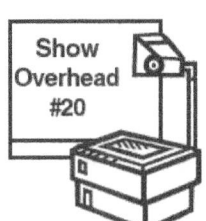

Round 4: Chris' Story

Read the story aloud:

Chris works for a city public works department. One hot afternoon the temperature outside reached 92 degrees. While Chris was shoveling dirt in a vacant lot, he started to feel dizzy and disoriented. He fainted due to the heat.

Ask the teams:

❝What solutions can you think of that might prevent this injury from happening again?❞

Have the teams post their solutions and compare them to the suggested answers below.

Remove the Hazard. Limit outdoor work on very hot days.

Work Policies. Limit outdoor work on very hot days. Have a cool place to go for frequent breaks. Have plenty of water available. Provide training on the symptoms of heat stress and how to keep from getting overheated. Work in teams to watch one another for symptoms of overheating (such as disorientation and dizziness).

Personal Protective Equipment. A hat to provide shade. A cooling vest.

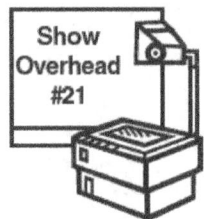

Round 5: James' Story

Read the story aloud:

James is a 16-year-old who works in a busy pizza shop. His job is to pat pizza dough into pans. He prepares several pans per minute. Lately he has noticed that his hands, shoulders, and back are hurting from the repetitive motion and standing for long periods of time.

Ask the teams:

> "What solutions can you think of that might prevent this musculoskeletal strain?"

> Have the teams post their solutions and compare them to the suggested answers below.

> **Remove the Hazard.** Provide a chair or stool for sitting while doing this task.

> **Work Policies.** Vary the job so no one has to make the same movements over and over. Provide regular breaks.

> **Personal Protective Equipment.** None.

Round 6: Maria's Story

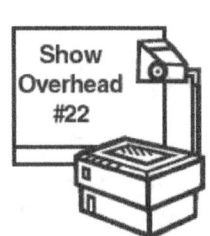

Read the story aloud:

Maria works tying up cauliflower leaves on a 16-acre farm. One day she was sent into the field too soon after it had been sprayed. No one told her that the moisture on the plants was a highly toxic pesticide. Soon after she began to work, Maria's arms and legs started shaking. When she stood up, she got dizzy and stumbled. She was taken by other farmworkers to a nearby clinic. Three weeks later she continues to have headaches, cramps, and trouble breathing.

Ask the teams:

> "What solutions can you think of that might prevent this injury from happening again?"

> Have the teams post their solutions and compare them to the suggested answers below.

> **Remove the Hazard.** Use pesticide-free farming methods. Or use a less toxic pesticide.

Work Policies. Wait the required number of hours or days after the crops are sprayed to re-enter the field. This should be on the label.

Personal Protective Equipment. Wear impermeable gloves and work clothes. If needed, wear a respirator.

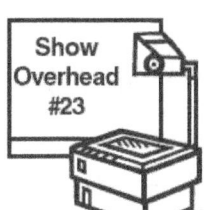

Round 7: Sara's Story

Read the story aloud:

Sara works as a nursing aide at a local hospital. She is expected to clean bedpans and sometimes change sheets, which requires lifting patients. Lately she has been feeling twinges in her back when bending over or lifting. She knows she is supposed to get help when lifting a patient, but everyone in the unit is so busy that she is reluctant to ask. At home, as she is going to sleep, she often feels shooting pains in her back, neck, and shoulders. These pains seem to be getting worse every day.

Ask the teams:

❝What solutions can you think of that might prevent this injury from happening again?❞

Have the teams post their solutions and compare them to the suggested answers below.

Remove the Hazard. Stop lifting alone. Lift patients only when other people are available to help. Or use a mechanical lifting device.

Work Policies. Make sure workers who have already been injured are not required to lift. Create a policy that workers may lift patients only in teams or when using a lifting device. Train workers about safe lifting methods.

Personal Protective Equipment. None.

Round 8: Brent's Story

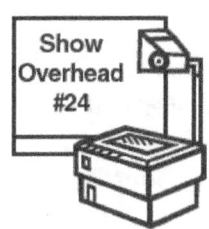

Read the story aloud:

Seventeen-year-old Brent worked after school in his father's pallet making business. One day Brent was working on a machine that helps take old pallets apart by cutting through wood and nails. The machine sorts out the old nails into a bin and then cuts the remaining wood into small pieces that can be ground into shavings. Brent's sleeve got caught in the mechanism of the saw. Before he realized what was happening, his arm was cut off. He was rushed to the hospital, but the arm could not be saved.

Ask the teams:

❝What solutions can you think of that might prevent this injury from happening again?❞

Have the teams post their solutions and compare them to the suggested answers below.

Remove the Hazard. There should be a guard on the machine to protect body parts from the moving parts of the machine. There should be an emergency shut off button in reach of the operator. The machine might be designed so the operator has to keep both hands on the controls. This would keep hands away from the moving parts.

Work Policies. There should be a rule that no loose clothing may be worn around the machinery.

Personal Protective Equipment. None.

6. Tally the dollar amounts. Determine the winners and hand out prizes.

Instructor's Note. If you wish, you can give students more information on hazards found on typical teen jobs and possible solutions. Copy and distribute the optional student handout in Appendix A.

C. Health and safety info search.
(75 minutes)

Note: The following activity may work best as a homework assignment which you may assign to individuals or to small groups. If your students do not have access to the internet, you may need to extend the timeframe to give them time to phone three agencies or organizations, request information, and have the information mailed to them.

1. Explain that in this activity students will learn how to find information on workplace health and safety hazards and effective ways to deal with them.

Ask the class to think about where they would try to find information if they wanted to know about a particular health and safety problem at work. Suggest examples of problems they might want to find out about, such as wrist pain when using a computer, or the hazards of a certain chemical. For each example you give, have students call out possible sources of information and write them on the board. Your list may include the following:

Sources in the workplace:

- Employer or supervisor

- Co-workers

- Union shop steward

- MSDS (Material Safety Data Sheet) for information on a chemical

- Labels and warning signs

- Employee orientation manual or other training materials

- Written instructions for work tasks and procedures.

Sources outside the workplace:

- Parents or teachers

- Internet search

- Government agencies such as OSHA, NIOSH, EPA, your state agencies, and your local health department

- Labor unions

- Community organizations

- Workers' compensation insurance companies

- Employer groups or trade associations

- University occupational and environmental health programs

- Professional health and safety groups

- Doctors, nurses, or other health care providers.

2. Explain that students will work in groups to see what information they can find about a specific problem in one workplace. We will focus on information you can get outside the workplace.

3. Divide the class into groups of 4 or 5 students each. Pass out a copy of Student Handout #7 to each student. Assign a different scenario on the handout (A-F) to each group. Tell them they have 30 minutes to research their health and safety problem. They must use at least three different

sources of information. These must include at least one government agency, and at least one organization that is not part of the government. They must complete all seven questions in part A of the handout (the Worksheet). Some suggested websites and phone numbers appear in part B of the handout (pages 3 and 4). In many cases the weblinks provided will take them directly to lists of factsheets on specific hazards. Each group should select someone to report back later to the whole class on what they found.

For this activity, you will need to arrange for the class to have access to a computer with internet connection, a telephone, or both.

4. After each group has done its research and completed its worksheet, bring the class back together. Ask each group's reporter to briefly describe what they found. Hold a short discussion on which sources of information they found most useful, and why. Make sure the points below each story are addressed during the discussion. If necessary, add them yourself.

Scenario A: Big Box Foods

Kevin works in a warehouse. He's seventeen years old. One day, when he was unloading 40-pound boxes from a wooden pallet, he suddenly felt a sharp pain in his lower back. He had to stay out of work for a week to recover, and his back still hurts sometimes. He is worried about re-injuring his back, and tries to be careful, but he wants to find out more about safe lifting and other ways to prevent back injuries.

What is the health and safety problem (hazard) in your scenario?

- Heavy boxes.

What information might you be able to get at the workplace? Where would you get it?

- Get training on proper lifting from the supervisor or a co-worker.

- Get written lifting guidelines from the employer or supervisor.

- Ask for information on available mechanical lifting devices.

What are the short-term health effects?

- Sprain, strain, or muscle tear.

What are the long-term health effects?

- Pain.

- Restricted movement.

- Difficulty in concentrating due to pain.

- Nerve damage.

- Weakness.

- Proneness to re-injury.

What are some possible solutions?

- Use a spring-loaded or hydraulic pallet that rises as boxes are removed (keeps boxes at waist height).

- Use a forklift or similar equipment so loads don't have to be handled manually. The driver of the forklift MUST be at least 18 years old!

- Decrease weight of boxes.

- Get training on safe lifting.

- Ask for help in lifting.

Scenario B: Brian's Computer Station

Brian has been working for six months as an administrative assistant in a large office. He is the newest employee in the office, and seems to have all the hand-me-down equipment. His keyboard and mouse sit right on his desktop, along with his computer monitor. The lever to adjust the height of his chair doesn't work any more. He works at his computer most of the day. He knows at least one person in the office who wears braces on her wrists because they are tender and painful, and who can no longer do a lot of things at home because her grip is so weak. Brian doesn't want to develop any problems like that, and wants to find out what he can do.

What is the health and safety problem (hazard) in your scenario?

- Repetitive stress at keyboard.

What information might you be able to get at the workplace? Where would you get it?

- Get training and help in setting up the workstation from the supervisor or a co-worker.

- Ask another injured worker what she's learned about prevention.

- Get written guidelines for ergonomic setup of computer workstations from the employer or supervisor.

What are the short-term health effects?

- Wrist pain.

- Numbness or tingling.

- Redness and swelling.

What are the long-term health effects?

- Carpal tunnel syndrome.

- Tendinitis.

- Decreased joint motion.

- Inflamed joints.

- Prolonged ache, pain, numbness, tingling, or burning sensation.

What are some possible solutions?

- Take frequent breaks ("micro" breaks every ten minutes; 5–10 minute breaks every hour).

- Make sure posture and position of body at workstation are correct.

- Evaluate the workstation, equipment, and furniture. They should support ergonomically correct postures. Look at chair design and height, computer screen height, keyboard height, lighting, glare, and clutter.

- Make sure job demands are reasonable.

- Do exercises to relieve physical stress and strain.

Scenario C: Dangerous Paint Stripper

Jessica has a summer job working for the city parks program. She has been using a cleaner called "Graffiti Gone" to remove graffiti from the bathrooms. She has to take a lot of breaks, because the chemical makes her throat burn. It also makes her feel dizzy sometimes, especially when the bathrooms don't have very many windows. On the label, she sees that the cleaner has methylene chloride in it. She feels like she's managing to get the work done, but she is worried about feeling dizzy. She wants to find out more about this chemical, what harm it can cause, and whether there are safer ways to do this work.

What is the health and safety problem (hazard) in your scenario?

- Exposure to methylene chloride in the paint stripper.

What information might you be able to get at the workplace? Where would you get it?

- Ask the supervisor or employer for a Material Safety Data Sheet (MSDS).

- Get training from the supervisor or employer on potential health effects and how to work safely with this chemical product.

What are the short-term health effects?

- Irritated nose, throat, and lungs, causing coughing, wheezing, and/or shortness of breath.

- A "narcotic effect" that causes light-headedness, dizziness, fatigue, nausea, and headache.

- Irritation and burning of the skin and eyes, with possible eye damage.

What are the long-term health effects?

- May affect the brain, causing memory loss, poor coordination, and reduced thinking ability.

- Liver and kidney damage.

- Bronchitis.

- Long-term skin problems.

- May cause cancer.

What are some possible solutions?

- Find a safer cleaner that doesn't contain methylene chloride.

- Use a respirator.

- Wear special gloves that are solvent-resistant.

- Wear protective clothing.

- Wear goggles or a face mask.

Scenario D: Noise at Work

Ediberto is 18 years old, and has been working for a company that manufactures prefabricated homes for about a year. He spends a lot of the work day using a power saw. His ears usually ring for awhile in the evening, but it seems to clear up by the morning. He is a little worried about whether it's damaging his hearing, but it's not that different than how his ears feel after a music concert. He wants to find some information on how much noise is bad for you, and what he can do.

What is the health and safety problem (hazard) in your scenario?

- Exposure to noise.

What information might you be able to get at the workplace? Where would you get it?

- Ask the employer for any noise level measurements that have been taken.

- Get training on hearing protection from the supervisor.

- Get training on OSHA noise regulations from the employer or supervisor. For example, noise from power saws may be up to 110 decibels (dBA). OSHA considers noise over 90 dBA to be hazardous and **requires** special protective measures. NIOSH warns that noise over 85 dBA is dangerous to hearing, and recommends that workers avoid it or wear hearing protection.

What are the short-term health effects?

- Temporary ringing in the ears.

- Temporary hearing loss (ears feel plugged).

What are the long-term health effects?

- Permanent ringing in the ears.

- Can't hear certain types or levels of sound, affecting your quality of life and enjoyment of hobbies. Often leads to varying degrees of permanent deafness that hearing aids cannot overcome.

What are some possible solutions?

- Find quieter equipment that does not generate hazardous noise.

- Use a muffler on the power saw to reduce the noise.

- Wear hearing protection when required (earmuffs are best, or use ear plugs).

- Keep workers away from noisy areas as much as possible. Limit the time of exposure.

- Get training on managing noisy tools and tasks and on how to use hearing protection.

- Measure noise levels and learn which are the noisier tools and tasks.

- Give workers medical exams (hearing tests) to monitor their hearing each year. Take action if they are losing hearing.

Scenario E: Needles in the Laundry Stack

Simone works as an aide in a nursing home. Her best friend's cousin Julia works in the laundry department. Simone has heard Julia complain about the medical staff, because used hypodermic needles sometimes show up in the dirty laundry. Simone is worried about Julia, but also doesn't think the medical staff could be that careless. She wants more information on what can be done.

What is the health and safety problem (hazard) in your scenario?

- Used needles.

What information might you be able to get at the workplace? Where would you get it?

- Get written guidelines for handling used needles from the supervisor or employer.

- Ask to see the employer's log of injuries workers have received from "sharps."

- Get training for all workers on proper handling of needles from the supervisor or employer.

What are the short-term health effects?

- Localized infection.

What are the long-term health effects?

- Hepatitis, AIDS, or other bloodborne diseases.

What are some possible solutions?

- Use needles with built-in safety features that decrease the chance of exposure, such as retractable needles. On some types, retraction is automatic and doesn't have to be activated.

- Use needleless systems for injections.

- Make sure sharps disposal containers are readily available.

Scenario F: Stop and Shop

Sarah works in a convenience store. She and the other employees take turns working the closing shift. It makes her nervous to be at the store by herself late at night, but she knows if she refuses the closing shifts, the owner will just look for someone else for the job. She carries mace in her purse, and the owner has told her to give up the cash in the cash register if she is ever faced with a robber, but she wants to find out what else can be done so she will feel safe.

What is the health and safety problem (hazard) in your scenario?

- Threat of violence from robbers or customers.

What information might you be able to get at the workplace? Where would you get it?

- Get training on how to respond to an incident from the supervisor or employer.

- Ask the employer for information on security measures that have been put in place.

- Ask the employer for information on previous incidents.

What are the short-term health effects?

- Possible injury.

- Stress.

What are the long-term health effects?

- Permanent injury.

- Death.

- Post-traumatic stress.

What are some possible solutions?

- Use safe cash-handling procedures (for example, locked drop safes and signs about limited cash available).

- Install physical separation from the public (bullet-resistant barriers or higher counters).

- Make sure visibility is adequate (good lighting, mirrors, signs kept low, windows unobstructed).

- Have rules about not working alone.

- Limit the number of unlocked access points (lock doors not in use).

- Use security devices (closed circuit cameras, alarms, panic buttons).

- Get training on handling emergencies, including how to recognize a potentially violent situation and how to respond.

- Consult with local law enforcement officials to develop a violence prevention program.

D. Review.
(5 minutes)

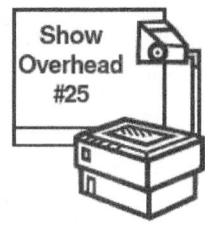
Show Overhead #25

1. Review the key points covered in this lesson.

    We've talked about how hazards can be controlled and injuries prevented. Remember that your employer is required under the Occupational Safety and Health Act to provide you with a safe and healthful workplace.

    It's best if your employer gets rid of a hazard completely, if possible. If your employer can't get rid of the hazard, there are usually many ways to protect you from it.

    In the next lesson we will talk about what to do in an emergency.

Tips for a Shorter Lesson

A shorter version of Lesson Three can be presented in 20 minutes by holding the discussion described in the Introduction and then reading aloud the stories in the *$25,000 Safety Pyramid game*. Brainstorm solutions to the problems in the stories.

1. **Introduction: Controlling hazards** (10 minutes). The class learns about ways to control hazards and prevent injuries.

2. **Work injury stories** (10 minutes). The class listens to real stories about teens who were injured at work (Overheads #16–24) and comes up with prevention strategies.

LESSON FOUR
EMERGENCIES AT WORK

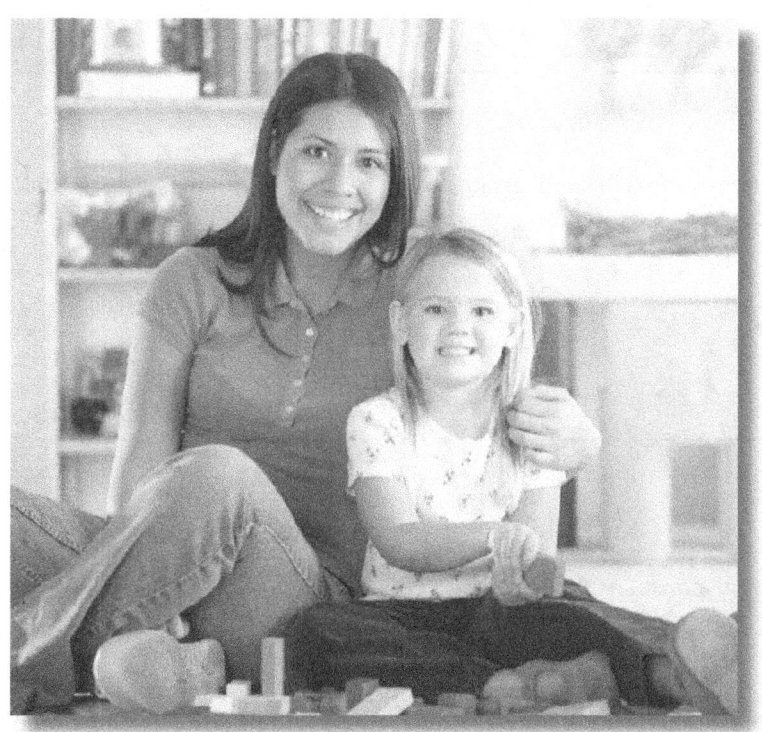

Learning Objectives

By the end of this lesson, students will be able to:

List at least eight types of emergencies that can occur in a workplace.

Explain what to do in at least three kinds of emergencies.

Identify important information employers should provide about how to respond to workplace emergencies.

Lesson Plan Four

	Activity	Time	Materials
A.	**Introduction: What is an emergency?** Students brainstorm examples of emergencies that could occur in a workplace.	10 minutes	• Flipchart & markers, or chalkboard & chalk.
B.	**Disaster Blaster game.** Students play a board game in small groups where they review what to do in various emergencies.	30 minutes	• Student Handouts #8–9. • One die for each table. • Game pieces. • Prizes.
C.	**Emergencies in the news.** Students work in small groups to evaluate stories about emergency response.	30 minutes	• Student Handouts #10–11.
D.	**Review.** Instructor summarizes key points of this lesson.	5 minutes	• Overhead #26.

Preparing To Teach This Lesson

Before you present Lesson Four:

1. Obtain a flipchart and markers, or use a chalkboard and chalk.

2. Copy the Overhead used in this lesson (#26) onto a transparency to show with an overhead projector.

3. For the *Disaster Blaster game*, copy Handout #8 (game board), one for each table of 4 students. Also copy Handout #9 (Disaster Blaster cards), one for each table, and cut out cards so that each table has one deck of 36 cards. Obtain game pieces, dice, and prizes, enough for each table.

4. For the *Emergencies in the news* activity, copy Handouts #10–11 for each student.

Detailed Instructor's Notes

A. Introduction: What is an emergency?
(10 minutes)

1. Explain to the class that we are now going to talk about emergencies at work. Tell students that:

   > *An emergency is any unplanned event that threatens employees, customers, or the public; that shuts down business operations; or that causes physical or environmental damage.*

2. Tell students that emergencies may be natural or man-made.

   Ask the class:

   "What are some examples of emergencies that occur in a workplace or that could affect the workplace?"

   Have students call out examples of emergency events while you write them on the board. Your list may include the following:

• Severe illness or injury	• Fires	• Floods
• Hurricanes	• Tornadoes	• Earthquakes
• Power outages	• Chemical spills	• Explosions
• Toxic releases	• Terrorism	• Violence

3. Tell the class that the best way to minimize the effects of an emergency is to know ahead of time what to do if that kind of emergency occurs and then practice the proper procedures. Few people can think clearly and logically in a crisis, so it is important to think through the proper procedures in advance, when you have time to be thorough and to practice.

When you start a new job, your employer should tell you what kinds of emergencies could happen in that workplace and what procedures you should follow to make sure you are safe. OSHA requires your employer to have an Emergency Action Plan which should include information on:

- What to do in different emergencies

- Where shelters and meeting places are

- Evacuation routes

- Emergency equipment and alert systems

- Procedures to follow when someone is injured or becomes ill

- Who is in charge during emergencies

- Your responsibilities

- Practice drills.

You should receive training about these things and participate in the practice drills. We will spend more time talking about emergency preparedness, Emergency Action Plans, and what you should expect from your employer. First we will play a game to see how much you already know about what to do in different kinds of emergencies.

B. Disaster Blaster game.
(30 minutes)

1. Divide the class into groups of four students and assign each group a table. Have them split into two teams. Pass out a game board (Student Handout #8), game pieces, a die, and one deck of *Disaster Blaster* cards (Student Handout #9, cut into 36 cards) to each table.

2. Explain the game directions. Tell students that the teams at each table should take turns rolling a die and moving ahead the number of spaces shown. They should follow the instructions written on the spaces for moving around the game board. Whenever a team's game piece lands on a square with a question mark (**?**), the opposing team picks a *Disaster Blaster* card from the top of the deck and reads the question to the other team.

3. Explain that teams may not always know the "right" answer to a question. Team members should discuss each question and use their best judgment. All players will learn the correct answers while playing the game. For each question, the opposing team reads the complete answer off the card after the first team provides their answer. If the team's answer is basically correct, they role again and their turn continues until they are unable to answer a question. If they do not answer correctly, they remain on the square where they landed until their next turn.

To win the game, a team must role the exact number needed to land on the Home Space and then answer a question correctly. If a team lands on the Home Space but answers the question incorrectly, they lose their turn and must wait until their next turn for a chance to answer another question. The first team landing on the Home Space and answering their question correctly wins the game. They receive a prize.

4. Tell teams to begin playing the game. Visit tables to check that students understand the instructions. Distribute prizes to winning teams or play non-competitively and reward all with candy or other prizes. Safety supply companies or fire stations may donate stickers, pencils, erasers, etc. with safety slogans.

C. Emergencies in the news.
(30 minutes)

1. Tell students that advance planning for emergencies is essential. It can reduce the risk of injuries or death. Your employer should have a written Emergency Action Plan and you should be trained about what to do in the different kinds of emergencies that could occur. Regular practice drills should also be conducted.

Ask the class:

❝What would you want to know if you were in an emergency situation at work?❞

Possible answers might be:

- What could happen in this emergency and how do I protect myself during it?

- Will an alarm alert me to the emergency? What does it look or sound like?

- Who's in charge during the emergency?

- Where do I go to be safe? How do I get there?

- If someone gets hurt, what should I do?

- Who in the building knows first aid?

- What are my responsibilities?

- How will I know when the emergency is over?

2. Tell the class they will next work in small groups to read news stories about emergencies that occurred at work, and learn how workers responded. In your small group you will read the story and decide what went well and what didn't go well. You will then list what should be done in this workplace to better protect and prepare employees for future emergencies. Groups will present their ideas to the rest of the class.

3. Divide the class into small groups of 4-5 students. Distribute copies of Handouts #10–11 to each student. Handout #10 is a set of news stories. Handout #11, Emergency Action Plans, describes key elements of emergency preparedness.

4. Assign a different news story from Handout #10 to each small group. Have groups select one person to lead their group's discussion by reading aloud their assigned story and the questions on the back. Another student should write down the group's responses to the questions. A third student may be designated to report the group's responses to the class.

5. Give small groups approximately 15 minutes to read their story and answer the questions on Handout #10. If they finish early, they may discuss the other news stories on the handout.

6. After 15 minutes, bring the class back together. Have the small groups report on their story, their evaluation of how the workers responded, and steps that could be taken in the workplace to better protect and prepare the workers.

Make sure the points following each story are addressed in the small group's presentation. If necessary, add them yourself.

Story A: Grease Fire in Restaurant Burns Employee

A fire erupted at Sunny's Family Restaurant Tuesday night, critically injuring an employee and causing $100,000 worth of damage to the building. The fire was caused when a frying pan, filled with oil heating up on the stove, was left unattended. The fire rapidly spread to dish towels hanging nearby. An employee discovered the scene and attempted to put out the fire by pouring water on the stove, causing the burning grease to splatter his face, arms, and chest. A co-worker, hearing the commotion, called 911 and yelled for everyone to leave the restaurant immediately. The fire department arrived, extinguished the fire, and attended to the burned employee. The victim was taken to Mercy Hospital and is reported to be in serious but stable condition.

What went right in this situation?

> The co-worker called 911 and yelled for everyone to leave the restaurant immediately.

What went wrong in this situation?

> The cook should not have left the stove unattended. Dish towels should not be located so close to the stove. It doesn't appear the employee who tried to put out the fire was trained. He should not have tried to put out the grease fire with water. A fire extinguisher or baking soda should be used instead. It appears there was no smoke detector or sprinkler system.

What steps should be taken in this workplace to make sure employees are better protected and prepared the next time?

> A smoke detector with an alarm and a sprinkler system should be installed. Employees should be trained about the hazards of leaving a stove unattended, what type of fire extinguisher to use, how to use it, and to immediately leave the building if a fire begins to get out of control. Once everyone is out of the building, the fire department (911) should be called. Practice drills should be conducted so everyone knows the evacuation route and where to gather to be sure everyone got out of the building.

Story B: Robber Threatens Young Employee With Gun

A 16-year-old employee of a local convenience store was held up at gunpoint late Thursday night by a masked man demanding money. The employee was working alone and in the process of closing the store for the evening. The employee later reported to police that, after emptying the cash register, the robber tied him up and then left with the money. Although the young employee was shaken up by the incident, he was not physically injured. The name of the young employee is being withheld because of his age.

What went right in this situation?

> The employee cooperated with the robber, which probably kept him from being injured.

What went wrong in this situation?

> The robber was able to tie up the employee and rob the store because security measures weren't in place.

What steps should be taken in this workplace to make sure employees are better protected and prepared the next time?

> Employees, especially young employees, shouldn't be working alone at night. There should be a silent alarm in place that would signal police or there should be a security guard. The store should be well lighted and have a security camera. All employees need to be trained in how to respond during a robbery or other threat.

Story C: Parents Praise Quick Action of Local Teen

Parents Charlene Cook and Kelly Nelson, who have children attending the Happy Go Lucky Day Care Center, called the Daily Times this week to praise the quick action of 17-year-old Tamara Thompson, one of Happy Go Lucky's star employees. Tamara noticed that an entire container of bleach had spilled near the janitor's closet and was giving off fumes in one of the nearby classrooms. Knowing that some of the children have asthma, Tamara walked the children to another teacher's classroom so they wouldn't be exposed. She then rushed back with paper towels to clean up the spill. Unfortunately, Tamara herself suffered breathing problems after cleaning up the bleach and had to be taken to the emergency room to be checked. She is currently at home recovering but plans to return to work when she feels better.

What went right in this situation?

> Tamara made sure the children were not exposed to the spill.

What went wrong in this situation?

> Tamara shouldn't have tried to clean up the spill herself, without being trained in how to do it properly and without the appropriate personal protective equipment.

What steps should be taken in this workplace to make sure employees are better protected and prepared the next time?

> Employees should be trained to leave chemical spills alone and to alert a supervisor so that someone with training and the appropriate personal protective equipment can handle it. Caution tape should be used to secure the area so others can't go near the spill. Personal protective equipment appropriate for the types of chemicals on site

should be available. In some situations, it is best to call the fire department to assist with spills.

Story D: Young Construction Worker Falls From Ladder

An 18-year-old house painter, who was painting the second story of a house, fell off his ladder yesterday, breaking both legs. He also suffered severe cuts when he caught his arm on a metal fence during the fall. Co-workers rushed to assist him and called for an ambulance. Local EMTs reported that the co-workers carried the fallen employee to the front lawn and then applied pressure to the open wound to stop the bleeding.

What went right in this situation?

Co-workers called 911. The co-workers knew to apply pressure to the bleeding wound.

What went wrong in this situation?

Employees should not have moved the injured worker because more damage may be caused. Only trained employees should administer first aid. It doesn't appear that the employees wore gloves before touching the bleeding young worker.

What steps should be taken in this workplace to make sure employees are better protected and prepared the next time?

Employees should be trained to call 911 or medical staff whenever there is an injury, and not to move a co-worker with possible broken bones because this can cause more damage. To stop the bleeding they should hand the injured worker a bandage to apply to his arm or apply pressure themselves using a thick clean rag. Workers should not leave an injured co-worker alone except to call for help. There should be a first aid kit easily accessible and several people should be trained in basic first aid. (Examples of items that should be in a first aid kit are bandages, antiseptic, aspirin/pain reliever, thermometer, latex gloves, sunscreen, tweezers, scissors, syrup of ipecac (to induce vomiting), sterile gauze pads, tape, and safety pins.)

Story E: 6.1 Earthquake Shakes Local High Rise Office Building

Office workers at R&D Business Solutions huddled under desks and doorways as a 6.1 earthquake shook their building. Once the tremors subsided, they followed lighted exit signs to the stairwell. They made it down ten flights of stairs and outside to the street. Gladys Royce, of Washington Township, whose son, Jason, is an employee of the company, complained that her son, who has Down Syndrome, was left alone to figure out what to do during and after the earthquake. The employees and supervisors had no idea Jason had remained on the 11th floor. The company pledges to take another look at its Emergency Action Plan and make sure the plan protects and prepares all their employees, including those who may need extra assistance.

What went right in this situation?

There were lighted exit signs. Employees took the stairs instead of the elevator. They didn't panic, so people weren't trampled. The company has a written Emergency Action Plan and will be making changes after evaluating what didn't work well.

What went wrong in this situation?

Jason was left alone rather than assisted to the staircase. It does not appear that Jason or the other employees received training or drills in how to respond in the event of an earthquake. It doesn't appear that there was a designated meeting place or a procedure for doing a head count to make sure all employees were accounted for.

What steps should be taken in this workplace to make sure employees are better protected and prepared the next time?

Employees should be trained to get under heavy desks for earthquakes. Practice drills should be conducted so everyone knows the evacuation route and where to gather so a head count can be conducted. Someone should be responsible for bringing the daily sign-in sheet to make sure all employees have been accounted for. The company should consider instituting a buddy system, or some other method, to assure that employees who need extra assistance are able to leave the building safely.

Story F: Tornado Breaks Windows at Local Department Store

A tornado blew through town yesterday, causing major power outages and damage to several buildings, including blowing out most of the windows in Johnson's Department Store on East 8th Street. As glass went flying, employees reportedly herded customers into the center section of each floor in the three-story building. Customer Tom Wilson expressed appreciation for the assistance employees provided in getting everyone away from the windows.

What went right in this situation?

Employees knew to get people away from the windows. Employees took responsibility for getting customers to safety.

What went wrong in this situation?

> The employees and customers should have gone to the lowest place in the building, preferably the basement.

What steps should be taken in this workplace to make sure employees are better protected and prepared the next time?

> Employees should be trained on elements of the emergency plan, such as going to the lowest level of the building during tornadoes or hurricanes and staying away from windows. Practice drills should be conducted so employees know the evacuation route and where to gather so a head count can be conducted. A supervisor should bring the workplace sign-in sheet to make sure all employees have been accounted for.

D. Review.
(5 minutes)

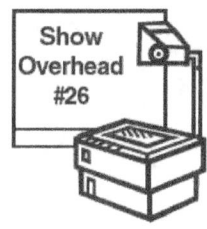
Show Overhead #26

1. Tell students that this concludes our lesson on emergency preparedness. Remember that every workplace should have an Emergency Action Plan. The plan should include the following information and workers should be trained about it: who is in charge during an emergency; where the shelters and evacuation routes are; where the meeting places are; what procedures to follow when someone is injured; where first aid kits are; who has first aid training; and how and when practice drills will be conducted. Tell students they are entitled to this information whenever they start a new job.

   In the next lesson, we'll talk about the right to a safe workplace, as well as other legal rights you have at work.

Enhancement Activities

◆ As homework, you may want to assign the task of creating something that communicates key emergency preparedness messages to fellow students similar to public service announcements students may have seen on TV. Examples include a poster, a rap song, a newspaper article, or a series of announcements over the school intercom system. Students may work individually or in small groups.

◆ An alternative activity is to stage a mock disaster using what are called "table-top" exercises or role play. Students are assigned a role to play (teacher, students, principal, parent, police officer, EMT, etc. and work interactively to act out a scenario. As the teacher you determine consequences based on decisions made by the student teams.

Tips for a Shorter Lesson

A shorter version of Lesson Four can be presented in 40 minutes by holding the discussion described in the Introduction, and then either playing the *Disaster Blaster game* or conducting the *Emergencies in the news* activity.

1. **Introduction: What is an emergency?** (10 minutes). Students brainstorm examples of different emergencies and discuss Emergency Action Plans.

2. **Disaster Blaster game** (30 minutes). Students play the board game in small groups.

3. **Emergencies in the news** (30 minutes). Students discuss the news stories in small groups.

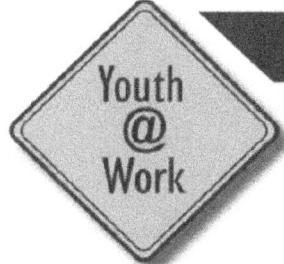

Youth @ Work

LESSON FIVE
KNOW YOUR RIGHTS

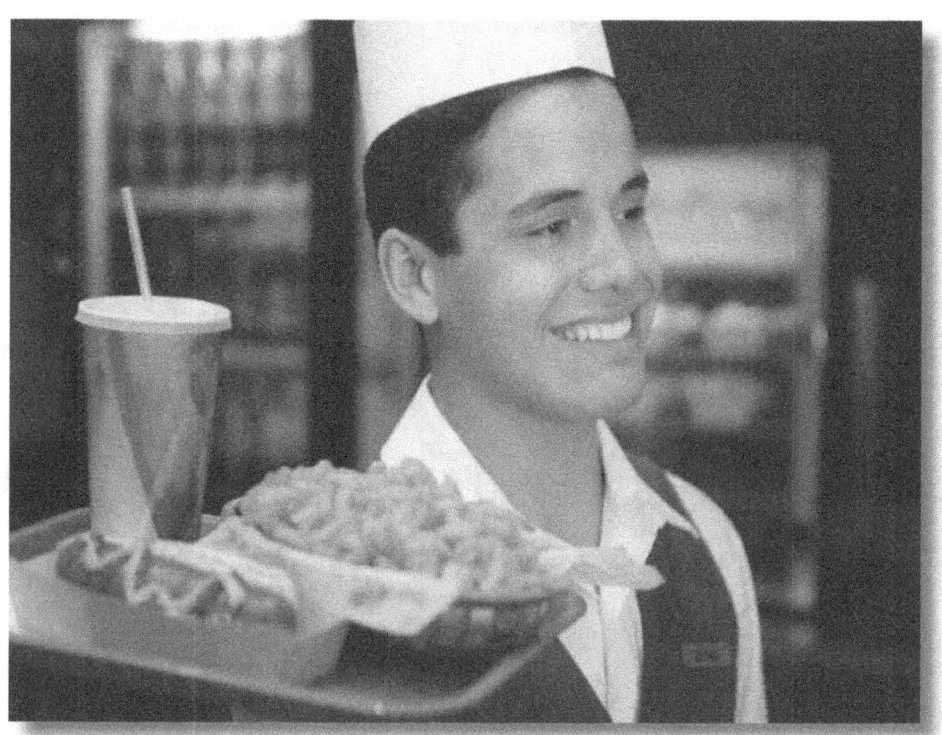

Learning Objectives

By the end of this lesson, students will be able to:

Describe the legal limitations on tasks that teens may do on the job, and on the hours they may work.

Identify two health and safety rights that teens have on the job.

Identify the government agencies that enforce labor and job safety laws.

Lesson Plan Five

	Activity	Time	Materials
A.	**Introduction: Your legal rights.** Students participate in a "warm-up" discussion to see how much they already know about teens' legal rights on the job.	5 minutes	
B.	**Review the factsheet.** The instructor points out where to find key information in the various sections of the factsheet.	5 minutes	• Student Handout #12.
C.	**Labor Law Bingo game.** Students work in pairs. They play a "Bingo" game to review information about safety and child labor laws.	15 minutes	• Student Handout #13 (set of Bingo boards). • Game pieces to use with Bingo boards. • Prizes.
D.	**"Jeopardy" game.** Teams review information about safety and labor laws as they play a simplified version of a popular TV game show.	30 minutes	• Overhead #27. • Prizes.
E.	**Review.** Instructor summarizes key points of this lesson.	5 minutes	• Overhead #28.

Preparing To Teach This Lesson

Before you present Lesson Five:

1. Decide which activities you will use to teach this lesson. We recommend you begin with the *Introduction* (A) and *Review the factsheet* (B). Then use **either** the *Labor Law Bingo game* (C) **or** the *"Jeopardy" game* (D).

2. Read the factsheet *Are You a Working Teen?* (Student Handout #12). Photocopy the handout for each student. The information in this factsheet reflects your state and/or federal labor laws, whichever are more protective. The more protective laws usually apply. Check with your state agencies listed on page 4 of the factsheet.

3. For the *Labor Law Bingo game*, use Student Handout #13, which is a set of 13 different Bingo boards. Have a board available for each pair of students. It is important to start by giving one pair Board #1, and then distribute the remaining boards in sequence to other pairs. If there are not enough different boards, photocopy more. It's OK for two pairs of students to have copies of the same board. Obtain game pieces to cover squares on the Bingo boards. These may be beans, pennies, or small pieces of paper.

4. For the *"Jeopardy" game*, copy Overhead #27 onto a transparency to show with an overhead projector.

5. Obtain prizes (such as candy) for the game activities.

6. Copy Overhead #28 onto a transparency for use in summarizing the main points of this lesson at the end of the class.

Detailed Instructor's Notes

A. Introduction: Your legal rights.
(5 minutes)

1. Explain to the class that teens have important legal rights on the job. Child labor laws protect teens from working long or late hours, and from doing certain dangerous tasks on the job. Health and safety laws protect all workers, including teens, from job hazards.

2. Ask the class the following questions to introduce the topic:

   ❝What is the minimum wage in our state?❞

Answer: See Student Handout #12 for the specific amount in your state. For your reference, fill in your state's minimum wage here: $_____ per hour.

"How late can teens work on school nights?"

Answer: Until 7 pm if you are 14 or 15, and until 11 pm if you are 16 or 17.

Instructor's Note: There may be exceptions for students in certain work experience programs. Check Student Handout #12.

"What agency can you call if there's a health and safety problem on your job?"

Answer: Call your local OSHA office. You can find your local office by calling 1-800-321-OSHA or visiting *www.osha.gov*.

3. If no one volunteers the answers to the above questions, tell the class the right answers. Explain that they will get more information on these and other legal rights in the next activity.

B. Review the factsheet.
(5 minutes)

1. Explain that students will now begin preparing to take part in a Bingo game. Distribute Student Handout #12, and ask people to look it over.

2. Point out the topics covered in the factsheet.

C. Labor Law Bingo game.
(15 minutes)

1. Explain that each student will work with a partner on this activity. Divide the class into "teams" of two.

2. Give each team one Bingo board from Student Handout #13. Also give each team a supply of game pieces. They will use these to cover the squares on their board as answers are called out.

3. Explain the game. The instructor will read the Bingo questions below. The questions are all related to job safety and child labor laws. After each question is read, students should call out possible answers. They may refer to Student Handout #12, the factsheet, to find the answers. The instructor should give the correct answer if the class doesn't come up with it.

Tell the teams that if they have a correct answer on their board, they should cover it with one of their game pieces. Note that some questions have several correct answers.

The first team to have a row of correct answers wins. The row may be horizontal, vertical, or diagonal. Everyone may count the center square of their board, which is a "free space."

At least one team will win by the time you've asked question #13. Give them prizes, then ask the teams to clear their Bingo boards and start a second game. Ask questions #14–26. When a second team has won, give them prizes.

Labor Law Bingo—Questions and Answers

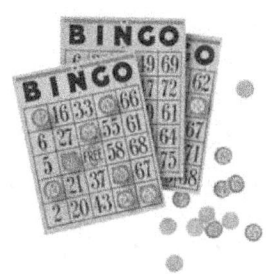

1. **What is the minimum wage in our state?**

   See Student Handout #12 for the specific amount in your state. For your reference, fill in your state's minimum wage here: $_____ per hour.

2. **Name one kind of machinery you can't use if you are under 18.**

   Meat slicer; fork lift; box crusher.

3. **How old do you have to be to do baking activities?**

   16 years old.

4. **Name a task that a worker cannot do until age 16.**

   Load or unload trucks; cooking; dry cleaning; work in construction; work in manufacturing.

5. **Name a task that a worker cannot do until age 18.**

   Roofing; driving as a main part of the job; prepare, handle, serve, or sell alcoholic beverages.

6. **If you are 16 or 17, how many hours can you work on a school day?**

   No limits.

7. **If you are 14 or 15, how many hours can you work on a school day?**

   3 hours.

8. **If you are 14 or 15, how many hours can you work on a Saturday or Sunday?**

   8 hours.

9. **If you are 14 or 15, up to how many hours can you work during a school week?**

   18 hours.

10. **Name one thing you can do to prevent a job injury.**

    Follow safety rules; get safety training; report unsafe conditions; refuse to do unsafe work.

11. **Under OSHA law, who is responsible for providing a safe and healthy workplace?**

    The employer.

12. **How late can 16- and 17-year-olds work on school nights?**

    11 pm. (This restriction can be waived with written parental *and* school permission.)

13. **Can a 16-year-old work in a dry-cleaning shop?**

    Yes.

14. **During the school year, how late can 14- and 15-year-olds work at night?**

    7 pm.

15. **During the summer, how late can 14- and 15-year-olds work at night?**

    9 pm.

16. **At what age do teens no longer need to get a youth employment certificate?**

    18 years old.

17. **Can a 15-year-old work on a ladder or scaffold?**

    No.

18. **How many teens in the U.S. go to a hospital emergency room each year for work-related injuries?**

    53,000 teens.

19. **In our state, where do you go to get a youth employment certificate?**

    www.nclabor.com

20. **What is the earliest that a 14- or 15-year-old is allowed to begin work in the morning?**

    7 am.

21. **What is the earliest that a 16- or 17-year-old is allowed to begin work in the morning?**

    5 am. (This restriction can be waived with written parental *and* school permission.)

22. **What is the name of the state agency to call about the hours you are allowed to work or the type of work you can do?**

    North Carolina Wage and Hour Bureau.

23. **What is the name of the state agency that handles complaints about workplace safety?**

    OSHNC—the Occupational Safety and Health Division.

24. **What is the name of the agency that handles complaints about racial discrimination or sexual harassment at work?**

    U.S. Equal Employment Opportunity Commission.

25. **What does Workers' Compensation pay for?**

    Medical treatment; lost wages.

26. **Name one health and safety protection your employer must provide.**

    Protective equipment and clothing; a safe and healthy workplace; safety training.

D. "Jeopardy" game.

(30 minutes)

1. Explain to the class that we will now play a game to review key information about health and safety and labor laws. It is based on a popular TV game show.

2. Divide the class into teams of 3 to 5 participants each. Have each team pick a team name. Write the team names across the top of the flipchart making a column for each team. These will be used for keeping score. The instructor can keep score, or can ask for a volunteer from the class.

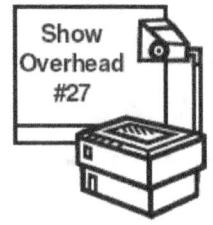

Show
Overhead
#27

3. Show Overhead #27, *Game Board*, and keep it on display throughout the game. Then explain the rules:

   - Teams may refer to Student Handout #12 to find answers.

   - The first team will pick a category and dollar amount from the game board. The instructor will ask the corresponding question.

   - The team gets approximately 30 seconds to discuss the question and come up with an answer.

   - If the first team answers correctly, they get the dollar amount for that question. The scorekeeper will record it in their column on the flipchart. Then the next team picks a category and dollar amount.

   - If the first team answers incorrectly, the next team in order will be called on to answer the same question. This will continue until a team gets the correct answer. They win the dollar amount. There is no penalty for incorrect answers. (Don't call on another team if the question is True or False.)

   - If all the teams miss a question, the instructor will give the correct answer.

   - Whether a team gets the correct answer or the instructor gives it, take time to explain the answer. Sometimes there are several possible correct answers, or more complete answers.

   - After a question has been answered, cross off that block on the game board (Overhead #27). Use a non-permanent transparency marker so the overhead can be cleaned easily.

4. Play the game. Proceed according to the rules above. At the end of the game, total up the dollar amounts each team has won. Give a prize (candy, etc.) to the winning team.

5. Questions and answers appear on the next page. If you need more information on these issues, see the *Resources* section at the end of the curriculum.

	Rights on the Job	Dangerous Work & Work Permits	Hours for Teens & Working Safely	Job Injuries & Getting Help
$100	True or False? Your employer can't punish you for reporting a safety problem. *True.*	How old do you have to be to drive a forklift? *18 years old.*	If you're 14 or 15, how many hours can you work on a school day? *3 hours.*	True or False? You can sue your employer if you're hurt on the job. *False.*
$200	What's the minimum wage in North Carolina? *$_____ an hour (fill in with information from Student Handout #12).*	Name one kind of machinery you can't use if you're under 18. *Power equipment (meat slicer, saw, bakery machine, box crusher).*	If you're 14 or 15, how late can you work on a school night? *7pm.*	True or False? Your boss can punish you for getting hurt on the job. *False—it's against the law for your boss to punish or fire you for a job-related injury.*
$300	Name two rights you have if you get hurt on the job. • *Payment for medical care.* • *May also get lost wages.*	If you're under 18 and still in school, what do you need to get before you take a job? *A youth employment certificate.*	If you're 14 or 15, how many hours can you work in a school week? *18 hours.*	What's the name of the agency that handles health and safety complaints? *OSHNC.*
$400	Name two health and safety protections your employer must provide on the job. • *Safe and healthy workplace.* • *Safety training.* • *Protective clothing.* • *Payment for medical care if injured.*	Name one kind of work you can't do if you're 14 or 15. *Baking, dry cleaning / laundry, using ladder or scaffold, construction, loading and unloading trucks, rail cars, or conveyors.*	If you're 16 or 17, how late can you work on a school night? *11pm.*	What agency enforces the laws about work hours and wages in North Carolina? *North Carolina Wage and Hour Bureau.*
$500	Name two rights all workers have on the job. • *To report safety problems.* • *To work without racial or sexual harassment.* • *To join a union.*	Name one kind of construction work you can't do if you're under 18. *Wrecking, demolition, excavation, or roofing.*	Name two things you can do to prevent a job injury. • *Report unsafe conditions.* • *Get safety training.* • *Follow safety rules.*	Name two things you should do if you get hurt on the job. • *Tell your boss.* • *Get medical treatment.* • *Fill out a claim form.*

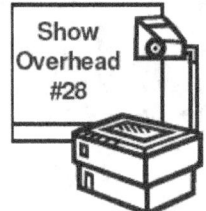

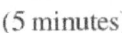
Show
Overhead
#28

E. Review.
(5 minutes)

1. Show Overhead #28 and review the key points covered in this lesson.

Federal and state labor laws set a minimum age for certain types of dangerous work. They also protect teens from working too long, too late, or too early.

OSHA says that by law every employer must provide:

- A safe and healthful workplace.

- Training on chemicals and other health and safety hazards at your job.

- Safety equipment that workers need to do the job.

OSHA sets basic workplace health and safety laws. You may have a state OSHA program which may set more stringent laws. The US Department of Labor's **Wage and Hour** Division sets and enforces minimum child labor laws regarding wages, hours, and prohibited occupations and tasks. Your state labor department may set more stringent laws.

By law, your employer is not allowed to punish or fire you for reporting a safety problem.

You also have the right to refuse to do work that is immediately dangerous to your life or health.

You can work more safely if you know your rights and responsibilities!

Tips for a Shorter Lesson

A shorter version of Lesson Five can be presented in 15 minutes by following the outline below.

1. **Explain the factsheet** (5 minutes). Pass out Student Handout #12, the factsheet, and describe the general content of each page to the class.

2. **Quiz the class using the "Jeopardy" questions** (10 minutes). Divide the class into several groups, and assign each group to read a page from the factsheet. Ask each group in turn a question from the corresponding category of the *"Jeopardy" game*. Rotate among the groups until you are out of time. Finally, review the key points of this lesson.

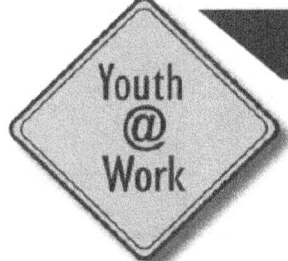

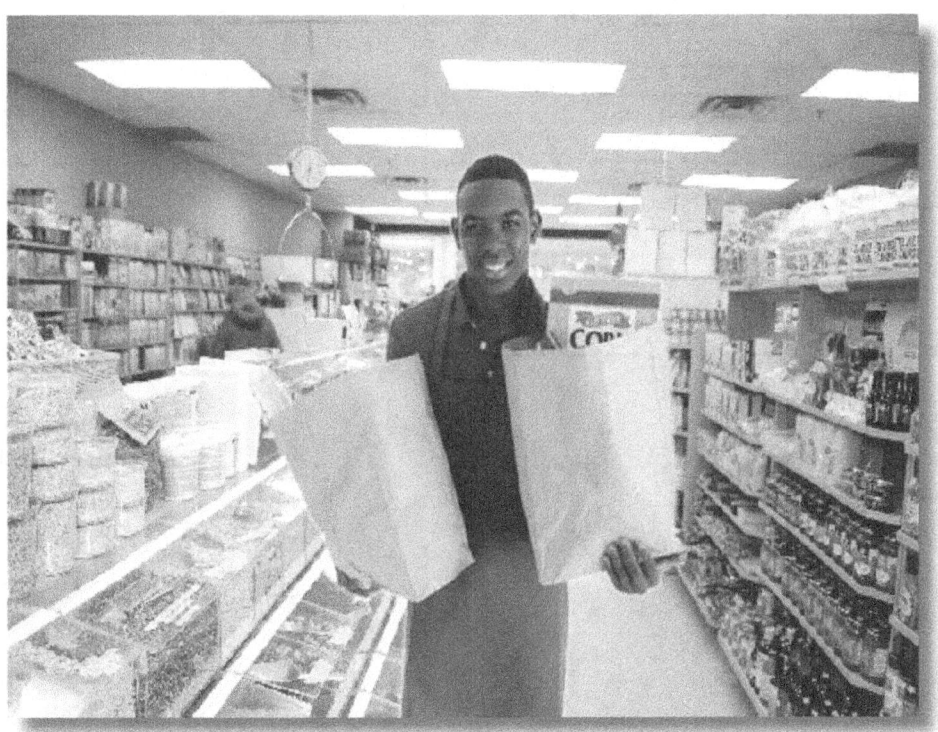

Learning Objectives

By the end of this lesson, students will be able to:

Apply safety and child labor laws to "real life" situations.

List three ways to get information and help on health and safetyproblems.

Discuss several appropriate ways to approach supervisors about problems.

Lesson Plan Six

	Activity	Time	Materials
A.	**Introduction: Steps in problem solving.** Instructor explains that this lesson is about taking action to solve health and safety problems and describes steps teen workers can take to address problems at work.	10 minutes	• Flipchart & markers, or chalkboard & chalk. • Overhead #29.
B.	**Mini-skits.** Students take turns enacting possible responses to health and safety issues at work.	20 minutes	
C.	**Role play: Elena's story.** The class listens to a realistic scenario about a teen worker in a sandwich shop and identifies violations of law. In small groups, students develop alternative endings for the scenario. Then groups role play the scenario, adding their endings.	30 minutes	• Student Handout #12 *(Factsheet used previously)*. • Student Handout #14.
D.	**Wrap-up and evaluation.** Instructor summarizes key points of this series of classes. Students complete an Evaluation Form.	10 minutes	• Overhead #30. • Student Handout #15.

Preparing To Teach This Lesson

Before you present Lesson Six:

1. Decide which activities you will use to teach this lesson. We recommend you begin with the *Introduction* (A). Then use **either** the *Mini-skits* (B) **or** the *Role play: Elena's story* (C). Teachers using this curriculum have found that, for some students, the Elena story presents too many issues at once, and that the mini-skits are more appropriate for these students.

2. Obtain a flipchart and markers, or use a chalkboard and chalk.

3. Copy the Overheads used in this lesson (#29–30) onto transparencies to show with an overhead projector.

4. Make extra copies of Student Handout #12, the factsheet, in case students haven't saved the copies they used during Lesson Five.

5. For the *Role play: Elena's story* (C), photocopy Student Handout #14.

6. Photocopy Student Handout #15, *Evaluation*, for everyone in the class.

Detailed Instructor's Notes

A. Introduction: Steps in problem solving.
(10 minutes)

1. Introduce the topic. Explain that the class will now learn and practice what to do when a safety problem comes up at work. They will also use some of the skills learned in earlier lessons, such as identifying hazards, controlling them to prevent injuries, understanding legal rights, and knowing where to go for help.

    It may be helpful to affirm to your students that young workers typically try hard to do a good job for employers. Unfortunately this can get students in trouble if the employer takes advantage of their willingness to do anything, even things that are not legal for them to do or for which they have not been correctly trained. Most employers won't purposely put students in danger, but there are far too many cases where employers allowed an eager young worker to do a task that was beyond his or her training. The results have been fatal. See the stories in Lesson 3 for examples.

2. First, ask the class:

> "Has anyone had *any* kind of problem at work, or a problem that someone you know has had, that you want to share with the class? It doesn't need to be a health and safety problem."

Then ask those who responded:

> "What steps did you or the person take to solve this problem?"

Ask the whole class:

> "What other steps do you think someone with this problem could take?"

As students answer, make a list on the board of the steps they mention. Although you will be listening to students' particular experiences when making this list, try to keep the steps you list general enough to apply to a range of possible problems.

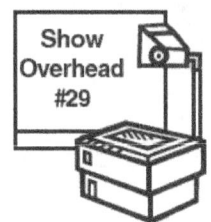

Show Overhead #29

3. Overhead #29 shows some of the steps involved in solving workplace problems (both safety problems and other kinds). Discuss these steps with the class.

Note to instructor: If you are doing Elena's story (Activity C) instead of the mini-skits (Activity B), you may want to wait to go over these steps until after students have had the opportunity to develop and demonstrate their own steps as part of the Elena role-play exercise.

- **Define the problem or problems.** Being able to describe the problem clearly is the first step toward solving it.

- **Get advice from a parent, teacher, or co-worker.** See if they have ideas about how to handle the problem, and see if they'll help. If there is a union at your workplace, you may also want to ask the union to help you.

- **Choose your goals.** Think about what you want to happen to fix the problem. You may want to write down your possible solutions.

- **Know your rights.** Be familiar with what hours you may work, and what tasks you are not allowed to do as a teen. Be familiar with your safety rights too.

- **Decide the best way to talk to the supervisor.** Figure out what to say and whether to take someone with you when you talk to the supervisor.

- **If necessary, contact an outside agency for help.** If you continue to have trouble after you talk to your supervisor, get help from someone you trust. If all else fails, you may need to call the appropriate government agency.

B. Mini-skits.

(20 minutes)

1. Explain the activity. Tell students that the class will be doing several skits about jobs in various workplaces. Explain that you (the instructor) will play the role of "boss" at each workplace. For each skit, you will ask a volunteer to come up and play the role of a "worker." You will present a situation involving health and safety, and the student will act out what the worker might say or do in that situation.

    Start with a practice role-play. Ask a volunteer to come up and help you demonstrate the practice scenario below.

    Instructor: You work at a grocery store as a bagger. I am the store manager. I ask you to help out in the deli cleaning the meat slicer. You've never done this job before and you are under 18 years old. What is the problem here? What do you say to me?

    Student (role of worker): I don't know how to do this job and I'm not sure I'm supposed to do it anyway, because I'm under 18. I'd be glad to help out in some other way.

2. Make sure students still have their copies of Student Handout #12, the factsheet used in the previous lesson. Have extra copies available. Tell them they can use these during the role playing if necessary.

3. Begin the role plays. Present as many of the scenarios below as you can within the time available. Ask for a new volunteer to play the role of "worker" each time you present a new scenario to the class. First read the scenario to the class and hold a short discussion of the issues it raises. Next have the student volunteer act out what they would say to you, the boss. You should then respond in the way a real boss might.

    After each scenario, ask the class if anyone else has something different they would say in this situation. Ask that student to come up and act out their response.

    Scenario #1: You work at an animal clinic helping to take care of the animals. I am your boss. I ask you to clean up one of the rooms that a dog has messed in. I tell you to use a powerful chemical solution on the floors and table tops. You have asthma and are concerned that the chemical may make it hard for you to breathe. What do you say to me?

    Scenario #2: You work in the warehouse of a hardware superstore. I am your supervisor. I tell you to pull items from the shelves to fill an order, but I talk quickly and don't make my instructions clear. What do you say to me?

Scenario #3: You work on the clean-up crew for the city's Parks and Recreation Department. I am your supervisor. One day it is about 95° outside and you've been working hard for several hours. You begin to feel really hot and tired, and worry that you might faint. What do you say to me?

Scenario #4: Your job is to shelve books at a bookstore downtown. I am your supervisor. It's 9:30 on a Wednesday night and the store is still very busy. I tell you one of the other workers went home sick and ask you to stay to help close the store at midnight. You are 15 years old and know you aren't really supposed to work that late on a school night. What do you say to me?

Scenario #5: Your job is to assemble parts at a local factory. You've heard that factories can be dangerous places, and it seems like there are a lot of hazards on your job. I am your supervisor. When you first started this job, I gave you some written materials on safety to read. But you are not a good reader and still have no idea what safety rules you are supposed to follow. Now I want you to sign a paper saying that you have been trained about safety. What do you say to me?

If you wish, you can create additional scenarios based on issues your students have faced on the job.

C. Role play: Elena's story.
(30 minutes)

1. Pass out copies of Student Handout #14, *Elena's Story*.

2. Ask for volunteers to play the roles of Elena, Mr. Johnson, and Joe. Have the volunteers come to the front of the class and read their parts aloud to the class.

> *Scene: Sandwich shop. Elena is a 15-year-old high school student. Mr. Johnson is her supervisor, and Joe is one of her co-workers. It is Thursday evening.*

Mr. Johnson:	Elena, Andre just called in sick so I need you to work extra hours. I'd like you to stay until 10 tonight.
Elena:	But Mr. Johnson, I have a test tomorrow and I need to get home to study.
Mr. Johnson:	I'm really sorry, but this is an emergency. If you want to work here you have to be willing to pitch in when we need you.

Elena:	But I've never done Andre's job before.
Mr. Johnson:	Here's what I want you to do. First, go behind the counter and take sandwich orders for a while. Ask Joe to show you how to use the meat slicer. Then, when it gets quiet, go mop the floor in the supply closet. Some of the cleaning supplies have spilled and it's a real mess.

Later: Elena gets the mop and goes to the supply closet.

Elena:	Hey, Joe! Do you know what this stuff spilled on the floor is?
Joe:	No idea. Just be careful not to get it on your hands. You really should wear gloves if you can find any. Andre got a rash from that stuff last week.

3. Ask students what laws were violated in the story. Suggest they look at Student Handout #12, the factsheet, if necessary. As volunteers answer, write their responses on flipchart paper.

Possible answers include:

- Elena was not given information about the cleaning chemicals.

- The employer didn't give Elena protective clothing (gloves).

- No worker under 18 may use a meat slicer.

- No one who is 14 or 15 may work that late on a school night.

- Some students may interpret Mr. Johnson's comments as a threat to fire Elena if she won't stay and work. An employer may not threaten to fire someone because they won't do something illegal.

4. Divide the class into groups of 3–6 students.

5. Explain that each group should come up with an alternate ending to *Elena's Story*, showing what Elena could have done about the health and safety problems. Assign each group one issue in the story to focus on (for example, working too late, working around chemicals, or using the meat slicer).

6. Encourage groups to think about these questions:

- How should Elena approach her supervisor about this problem?

- What are the different ways her supervisor might respond?

- Where else could Elena get help?

7. Groups may refer to the factsheet (Student Handout #12) if necessary. Explain that they will be role playing their alternate endings. They should assign parts, decide roughly what each person will say, and take notes if necessary.

8. After about 15 minutes, bring the class back together.

9. Ask several of the groups (or all, if there is time) to act out their alternate endings to the *Elena's Story* skit.

   Possible endings include:

   - Elena asks a co-worker, friend, parent, or teacher for advice.

   - Elena tells her supervisor she is uncomfortable with the late hours and prohibited duties.

   - Elena asks a union or community organization for information on workers' rights.

   - Elena quits her job because of the long hours or other inappropriate requests.

   - Elena refuses to use the meat slicer because, by law, she is too young.

   - Elena files a complaint with OSHA or the labor law enforcement agency.

10. Ask the class to comment on how effective each group's ending is.

    Questions to consider include:

    "How serious is the problem?"

    "Is it urgent to get it corrected?"

    "Will any of these approaches endanger Elena's job?"

    "Which approaches will be most effective in solving the problem?"

11. Review the problem-solving steps from Activity A, step 3 of this lesson.

D. Wrap-up and evaluation.
(10 minutes)

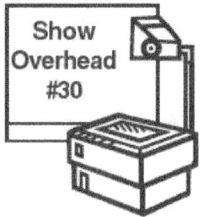
Show Overhead #30

1. Tell the class that this ends the last lesson of this introductory course on occupational safety and health. During this lesson we've talked about how to speak up effectively at work when there is a problem. It's important to know your rights, but it's also important to think through how you want to approach your supervisor with a problem. It's usually helpful to talk it over first with your parents, teachers, co-workers, union representative, or someone else you trust. If necessary, there are agencies to help you like OSHA or the federal or state labor law enforcement agency.

    Remember:

    *   Know your rights.

    *   Know your responsibilities.

    *   Know that your employer has a legal responsibility to keep your workplace safe.

    *   Know how to solve problems as they arise.

    Encourage students to ask their employers what the procedures are for bringing up problems they run into at work. If you are responsible for placing students in jobs, this may be a topic you want to raise with employers.

    Remind students that their employers have a responsibility to provide them with a safe workplace and to give them specific training about hazards on their job.

2. Pass out Student Handout #15, *Evaluation*. Ask students to complete and return it. They do not have to put their names on it.

Enhancement Activity

◆ Workplace harassment and discrimination are serious issues. You could have students visit the Youth at Work website of the Equal Employment Opportunity Commission, *www.youth.eeoc.gov*, for more information, as well as the agency that enforces discrimination laws in your state (listed in Student Handout #12). Students can test their knowledge on the "Challenge Yourself" portion of the EEOC site, *www.youth.eeoc.gov/scenarios.html*. Students could prepare written or oral reports, posters, or other forms of information messages regarding harassment prevention and resolution.

Tips for a Shorter Lesson

A shorter version of Lesson Six can be presented in 15 minutes by following the outline below.

1. **Read the skit** (5 minutes). Have volunteers read the class *Elena's Story* (Student Handout #14).

2. **List laws that were violated** (5 minutes). Ask the class to list problems they identify in the skit. They can use Student Handout #12 to help.

3. **Discuss possible approaches and problem-solving steps** (5 minutes). Ask the class what Elena could do to handle the problems shown in the skit. Explain the basic problem solving steps you want to promote. Finally, review the key points of this lesson.

John's Story

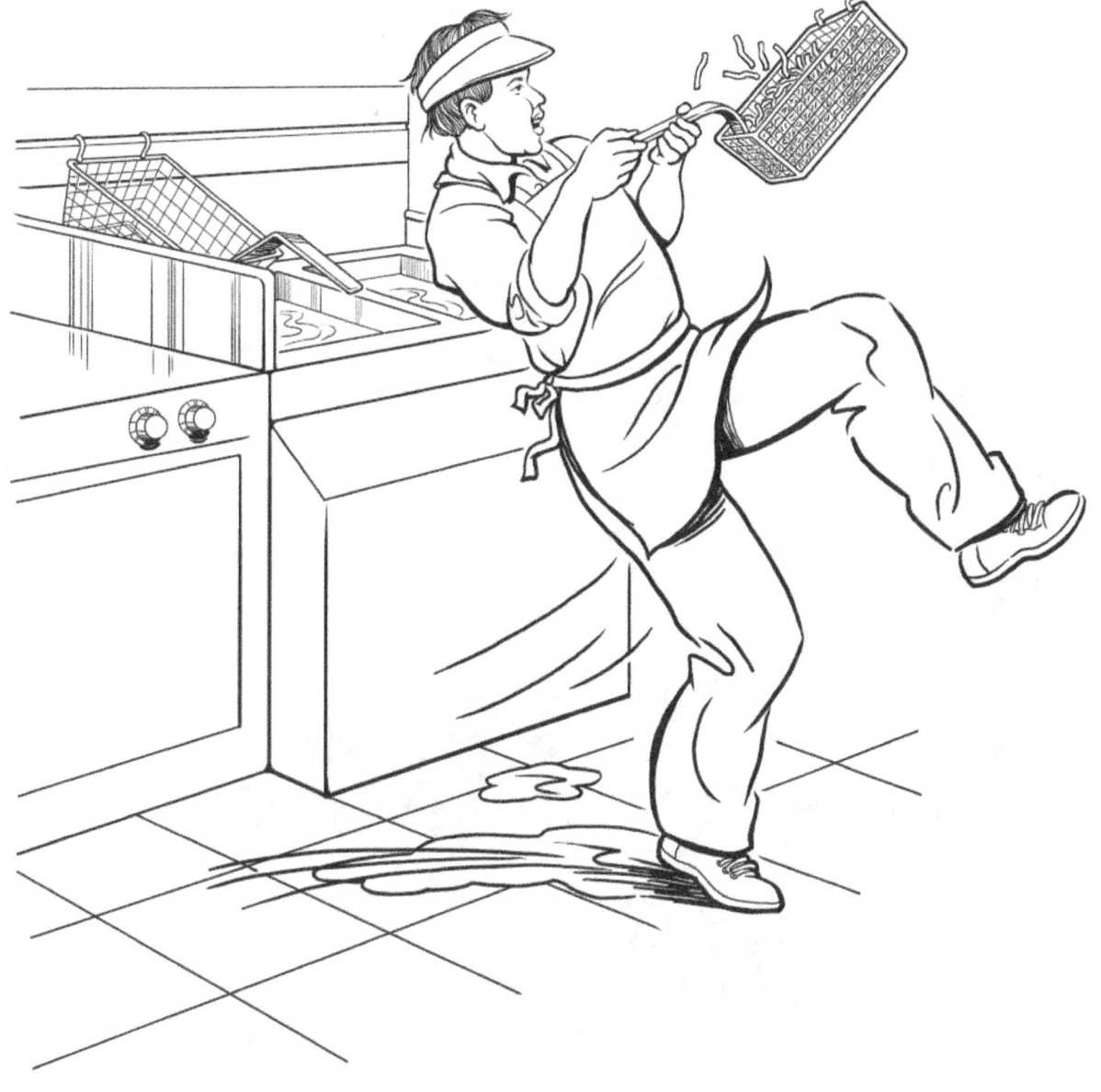

Job: Fast food worker

Injury: Slipped on greasy floor

Antonio's Story

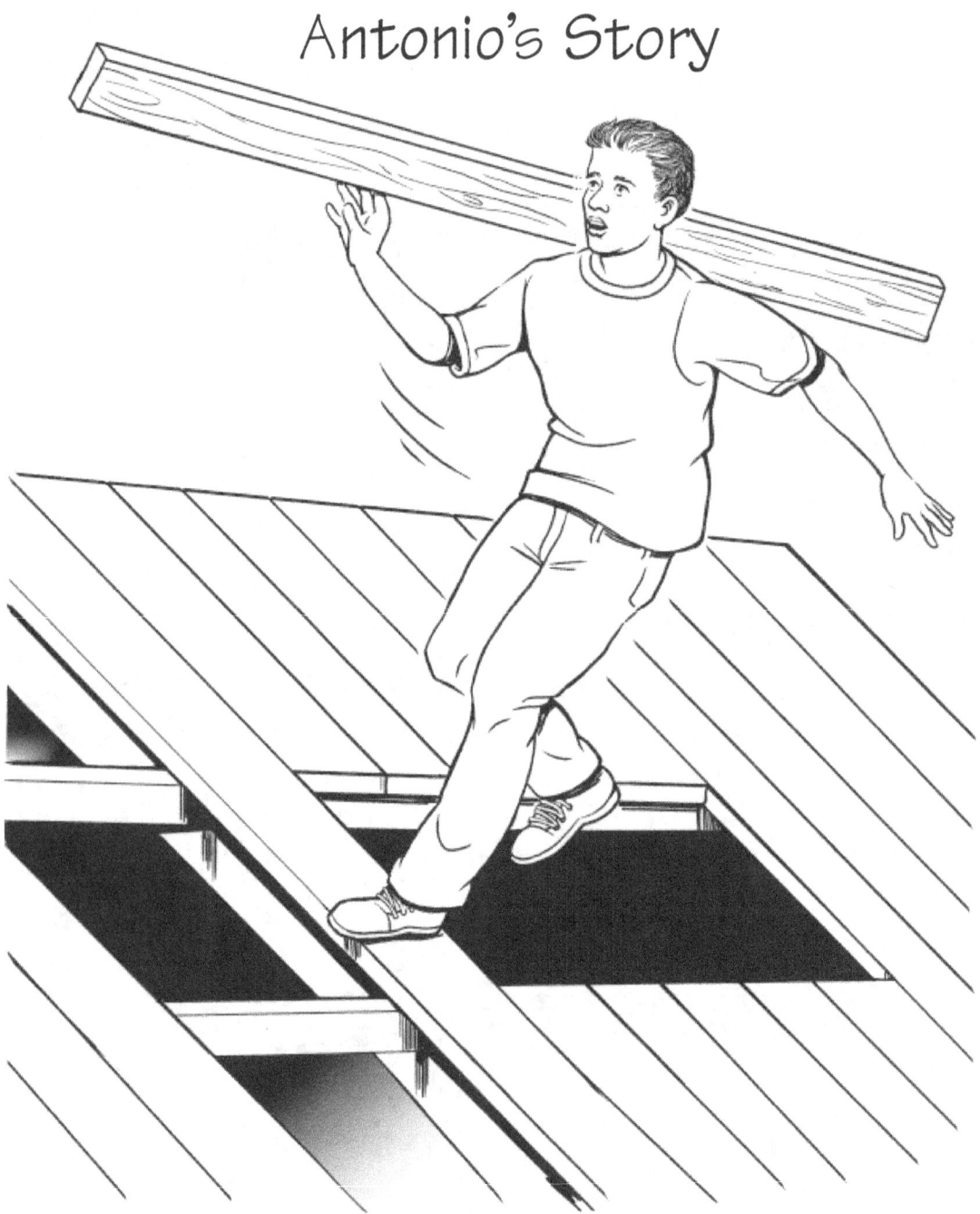

Job: Construction helper

Injury: Fell from roof

Keisha's Story

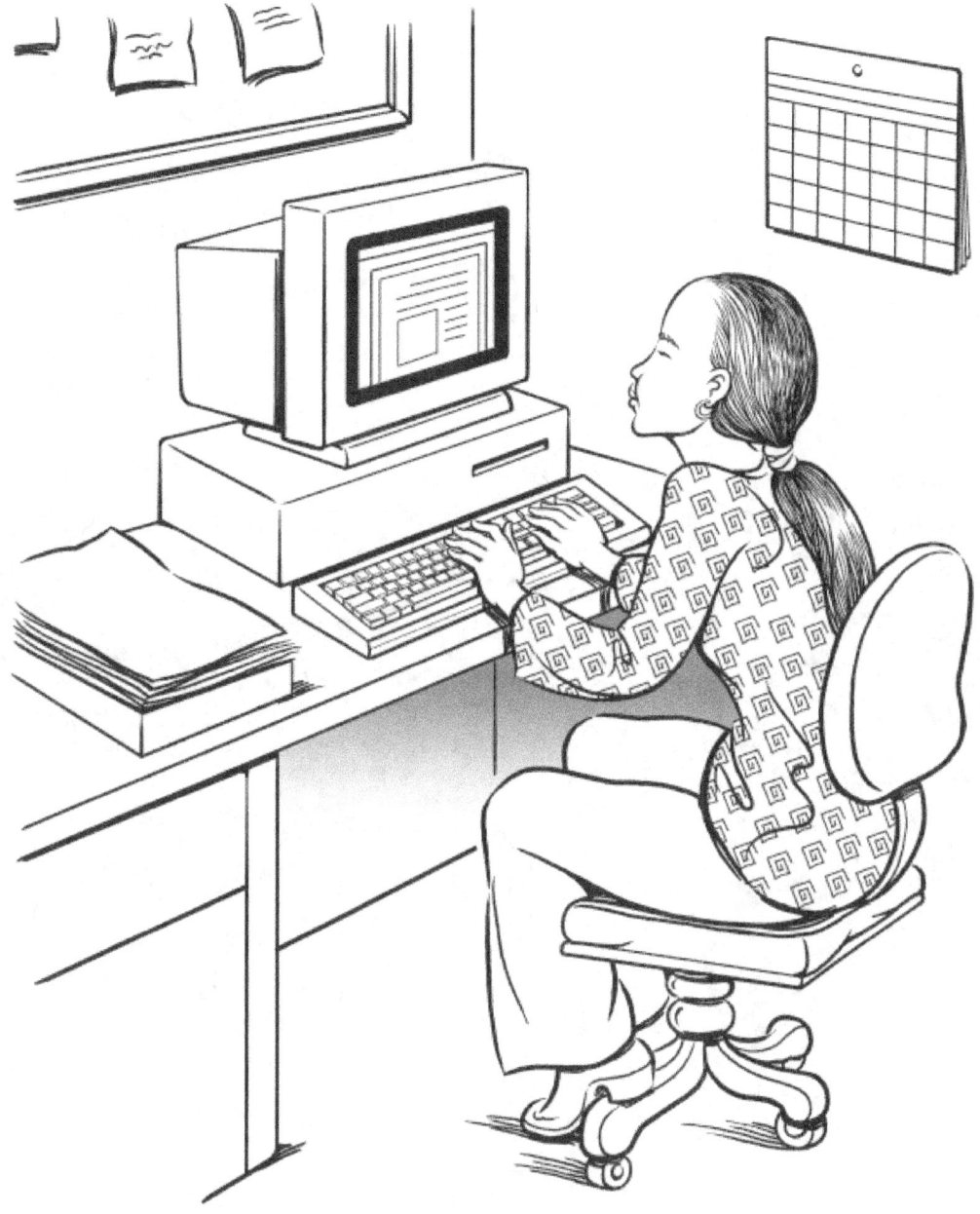

Job: Computer data entry

Injury: Repetitive stress injury

Francisco's Story

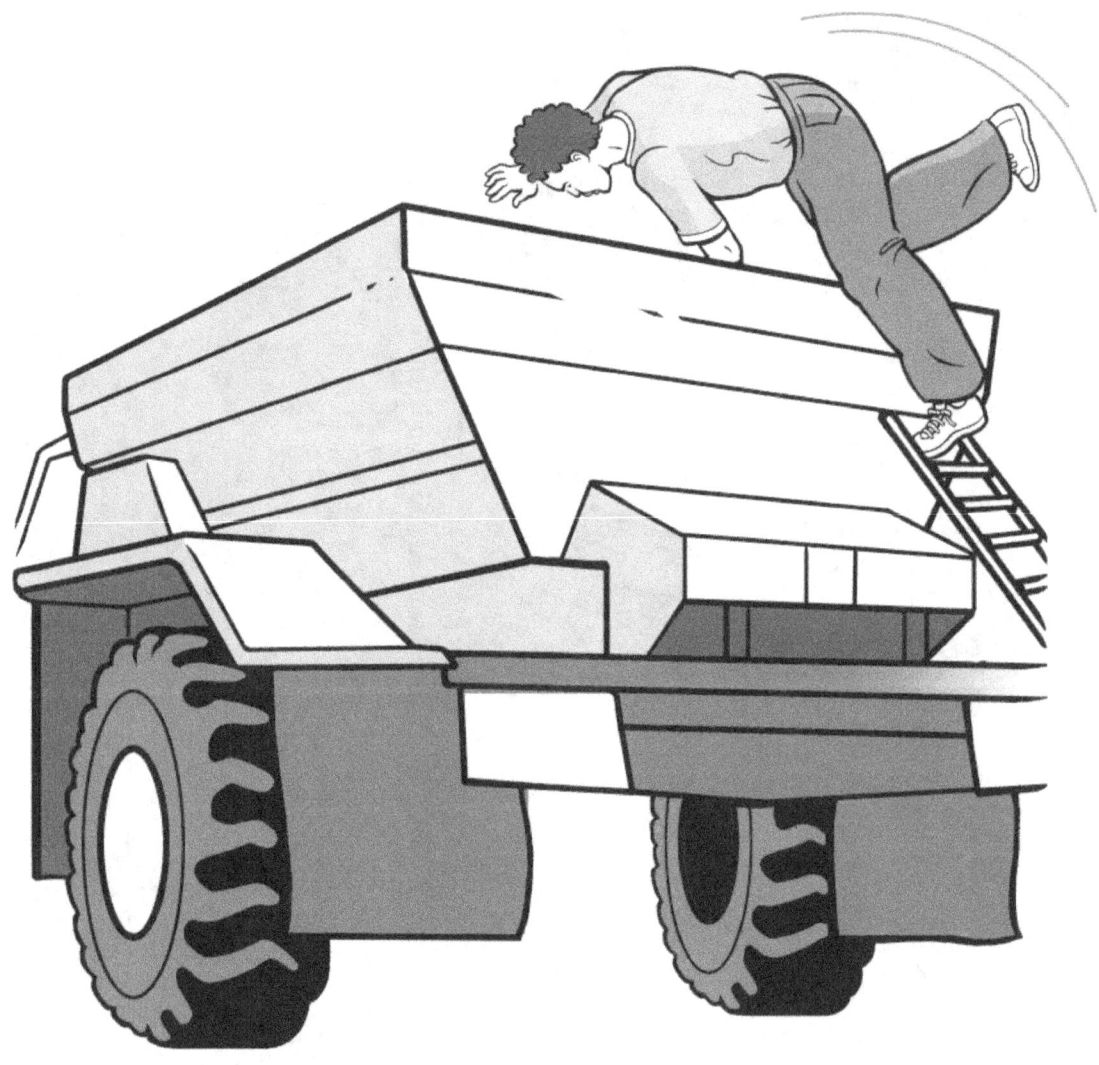

Job: Landscaping worker

Injury: Death

Where are teens injured?

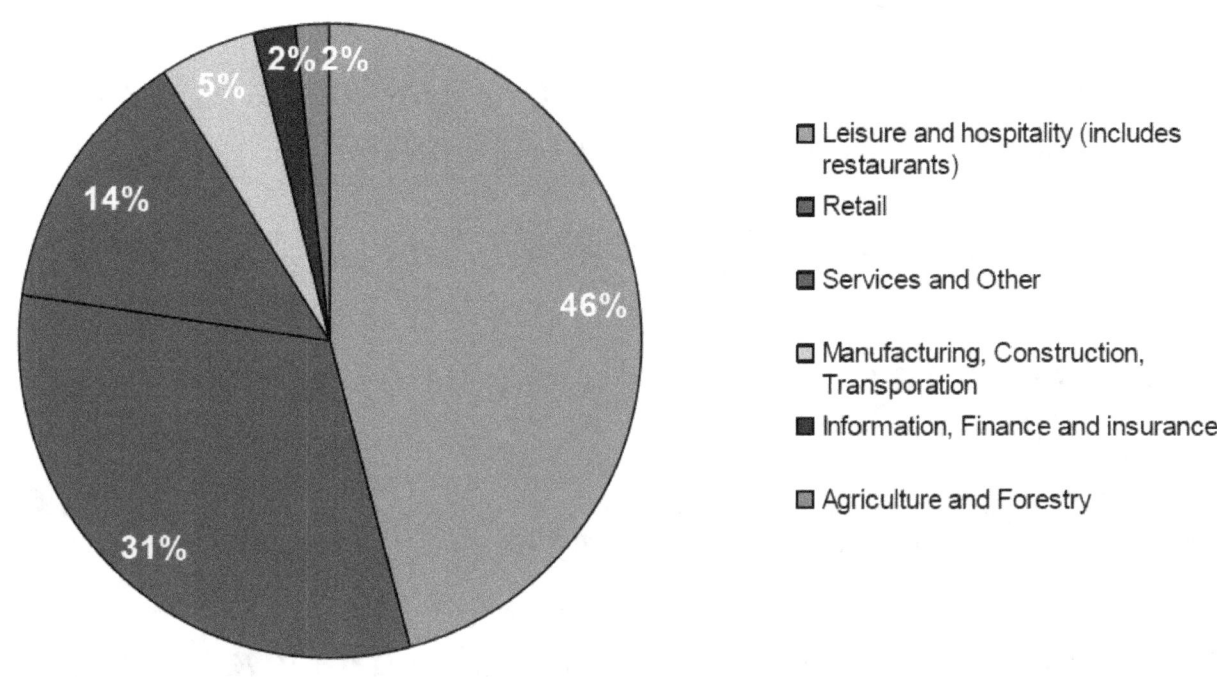

- Leisure and hospitality (includes restaurants)
- Retail
- Services and Other
- Manufacturing, Construction, Transporation
- Information, Finance and insurance
- Agriculture and Forestry

Where teens work

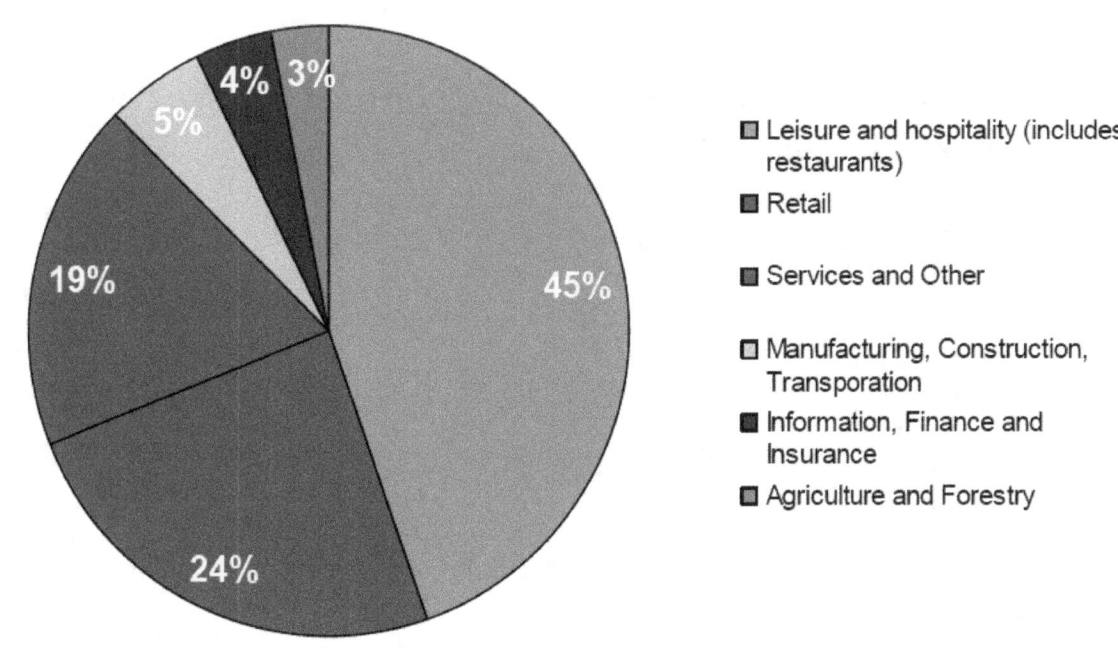

- Leisure and hospitality (includes restaurants)
- Retail
- Services and Other
- Manufacturing, Construction, Transporation
- Information, Finance and Insurance
- Agriculture and Forestry

Your Safety IQ Quiz

1. The law says your employer must give you training about health and safety hazards on your job.

   ☐ True   ☐ False

2. The law sets limits on how late you may work on a school night if you are under 16

   ☐ True   ☐ False

3. If you are 16 years old you are allowed to drive a car on public streets as part of your job.

   ☐ True   ☐ False

4. If you're injured on the job, your employer must pay for your medical care.

   ☐ True   ☐ False

5. How many teens get injured on the job in the U.S.?

   ☐ One per day   ☐ One per hour
   ☐ One every 10 minutes

Key Points of This Training

You will learn more about:

- Identifying and reducing hazards on the job

- Laws that protect teens from working too late or too long

- Laws that protect teens from doing dangerous work

- How to solve health and safety problems at work

- What agencies enforce health and safety laws and child labor laws

- What to do in an emergency.

Job Hazards

A job hazard is anything at work that can hurt you, either physically or mentally.

- **Safety hazards** can cause immediate accidents and injuries.

    Examples: hot surfaces or slippery floors.

- **Chemical hazards** are gases, vapors, liquids, or dusts that can harm your body.

    Examples: cleaning products or pesticides.

- **Biological hazards** are living things that can cause sickness or disease.

    Examples: bacteria, viruses, or insects.

- **Other health hazards** are harmful things, not in the other categories, that can injure you or make you sick. These hazards are sometimes less obvious because they may not cause health problems right away.

    Examples: noise or repetitive movements.

Find the Hazards: Fast Food

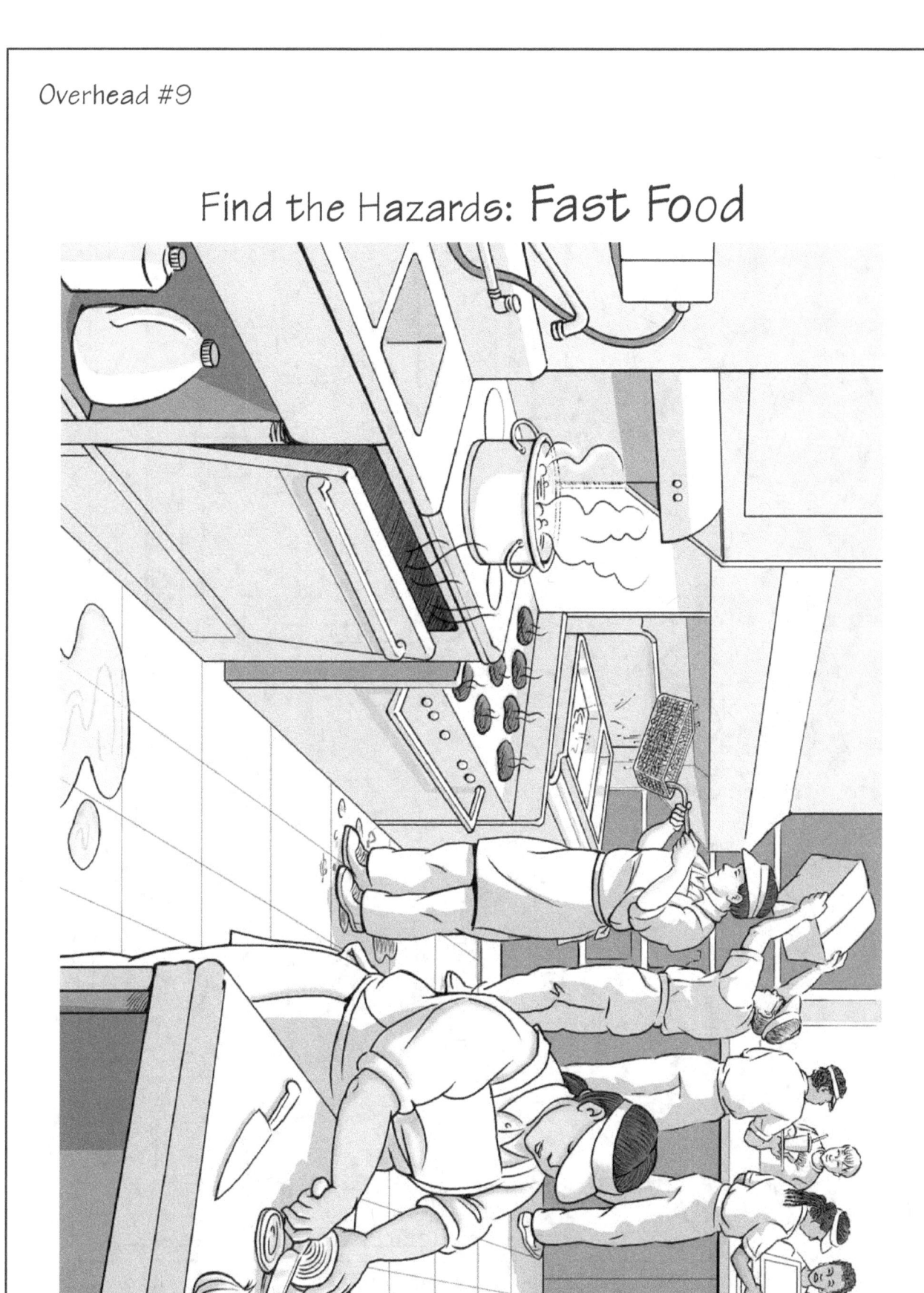

Find the Hazards: Grocery Store

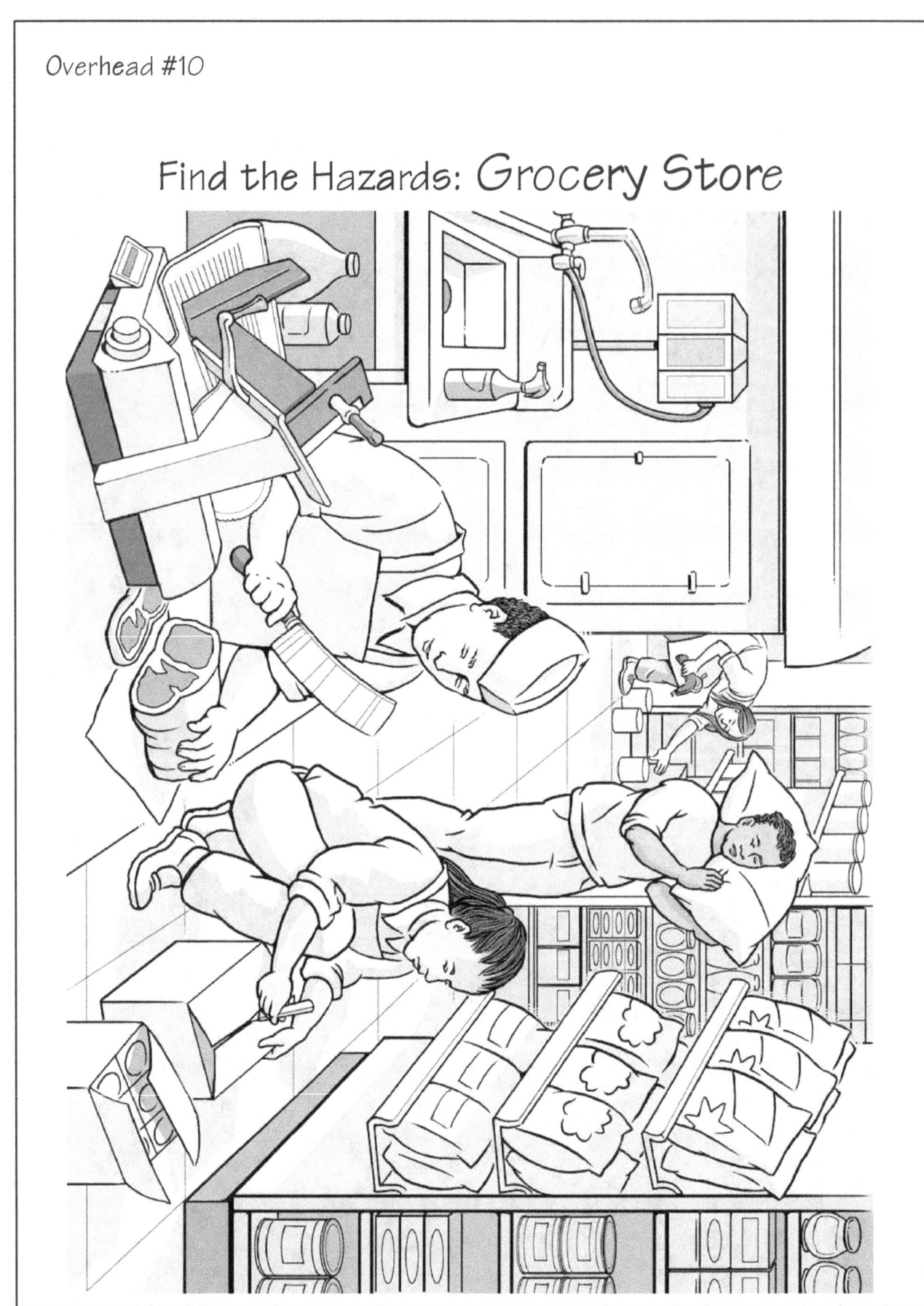

Find the Hazards: Office

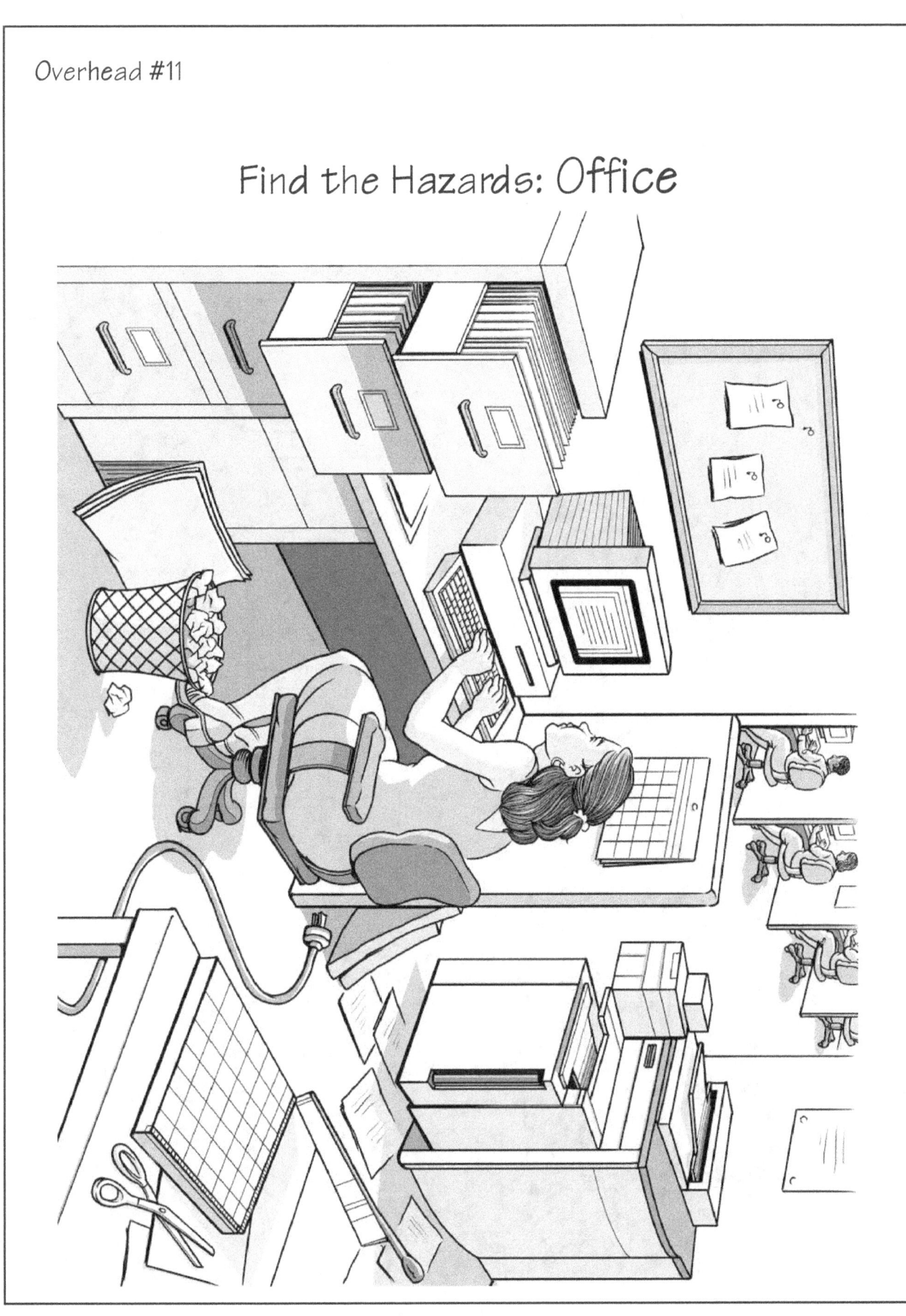

Find the Hazards: Gas Station

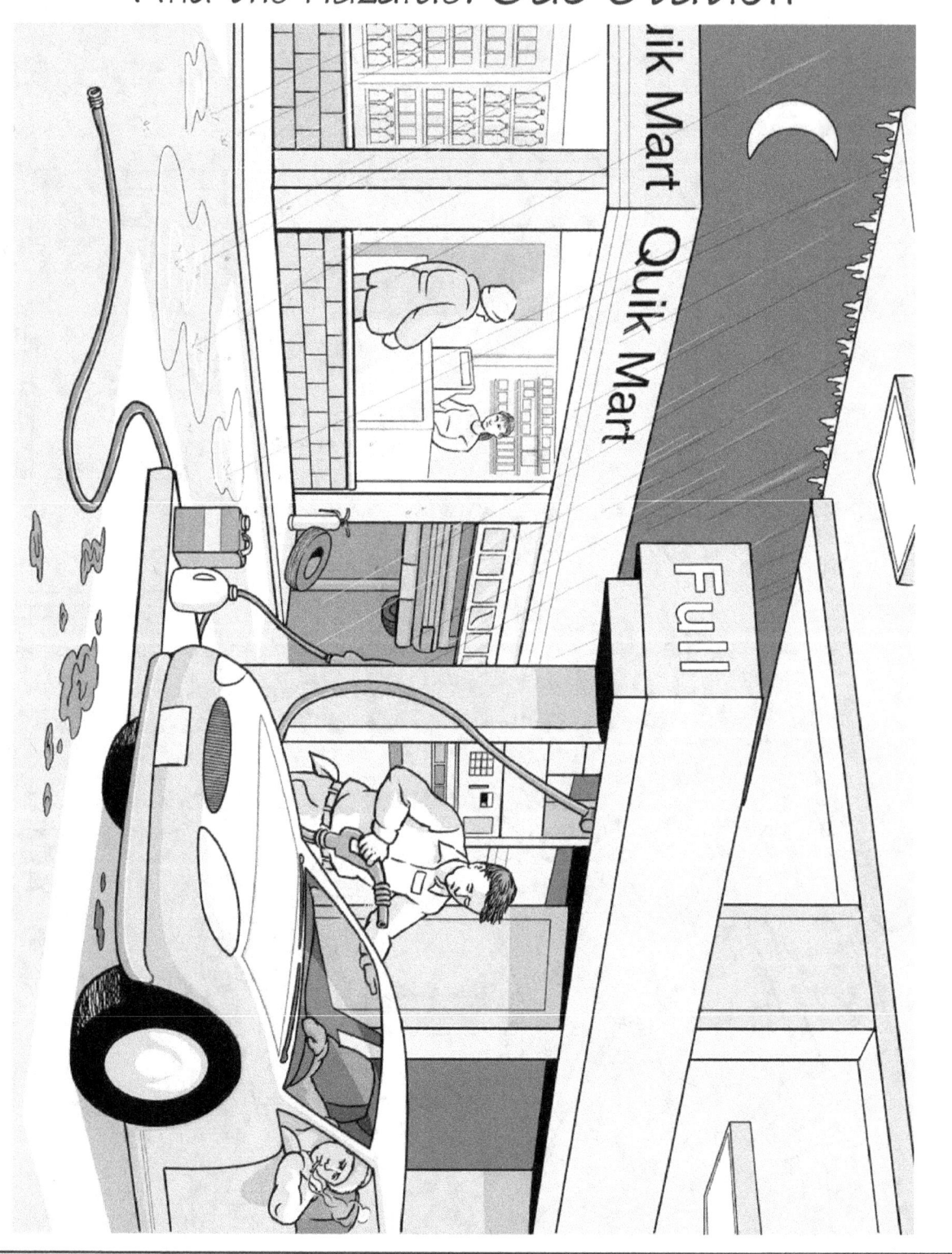

Sample Hazard Map

Students will draw maps in color:

Red = Safety Hazards   Green = Chemical Hazards   Orange = Biological Hazards   **Blue** = Other Health Hazards

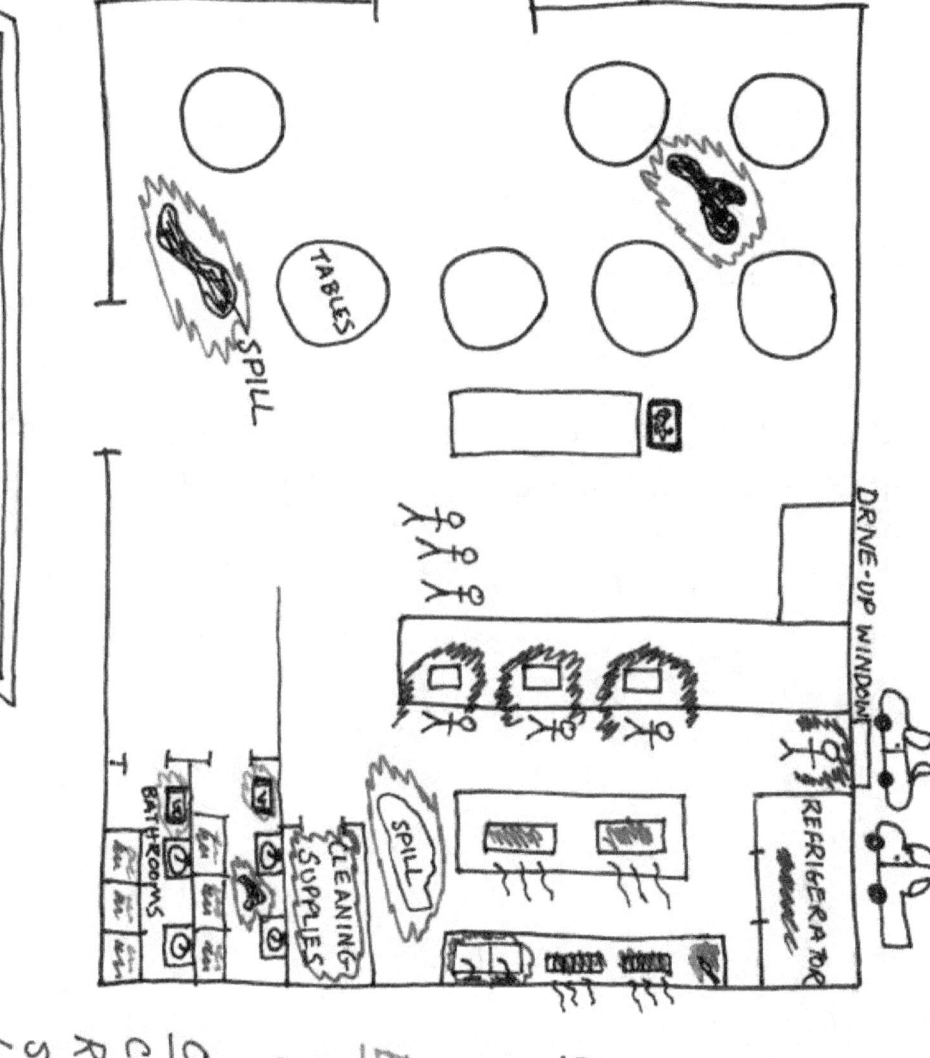

FAST FOOD RESTAURANT

TABLES

SPILL

DRIVE-UP WINDOW

REFRIGERATOR

CLEANING SUPPLIES

SPILL

BATHROOMS

SAFETY (RED)
HOT GRILL
HOT GREASE
SHARP KNIVES
SLIPPERY FLOORS

CHEMICAL (GREEN)
CLEANING PRODUCTS
DISHWASHING PRODUCTS

BIOLOGICAL (ORANGE)
BACTERIA
USED NEEDLES

OTHER (BLUE)
CUSTOMERS/STRESS
ROBBERY
STANDING
LIFTING

Key Points: Finding Hazards

- Every job has health and safety hazards.

- You should always be aware of these hazards.

- Find out about chemicals at work by checking labels, reading MSDSs, and getting training.

Controlling Hazards

First Choice: **Remove the hazard**

Examples:

- Use safer chemicals.

- Put guards around hot surfaces.

Next Choice: **Improve work policies and procedures**

Examples:

- Give workers safety training.

- Assign enough people to do the job safely.

Last Choice: **Use protective clothing and equipment**

Examples:

- Wear gloves.

- Use a respirator.

Jamie's Story

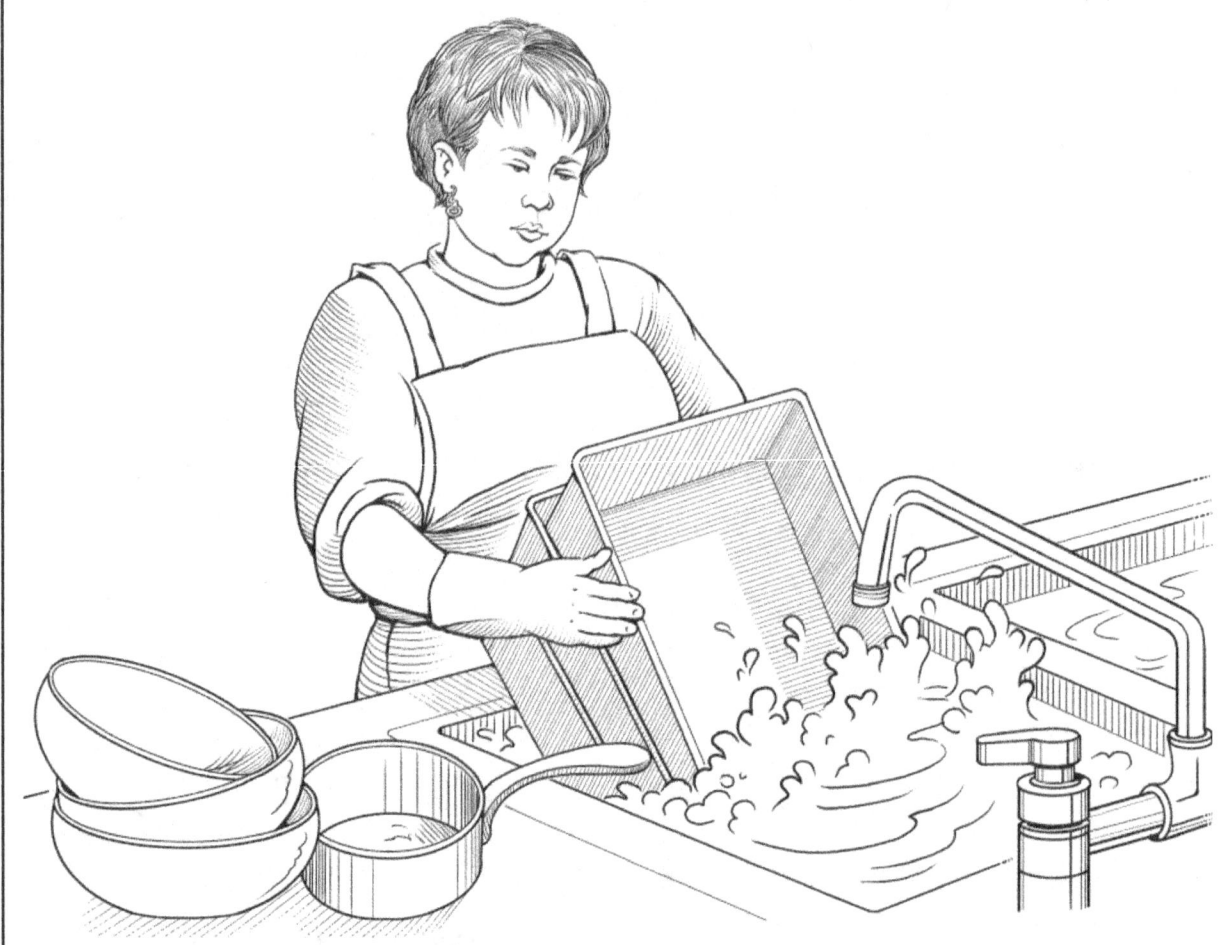

Job: Hospital dishwasher

Injury: Dishwashing chemical splashed in
         eye

Billy's Story

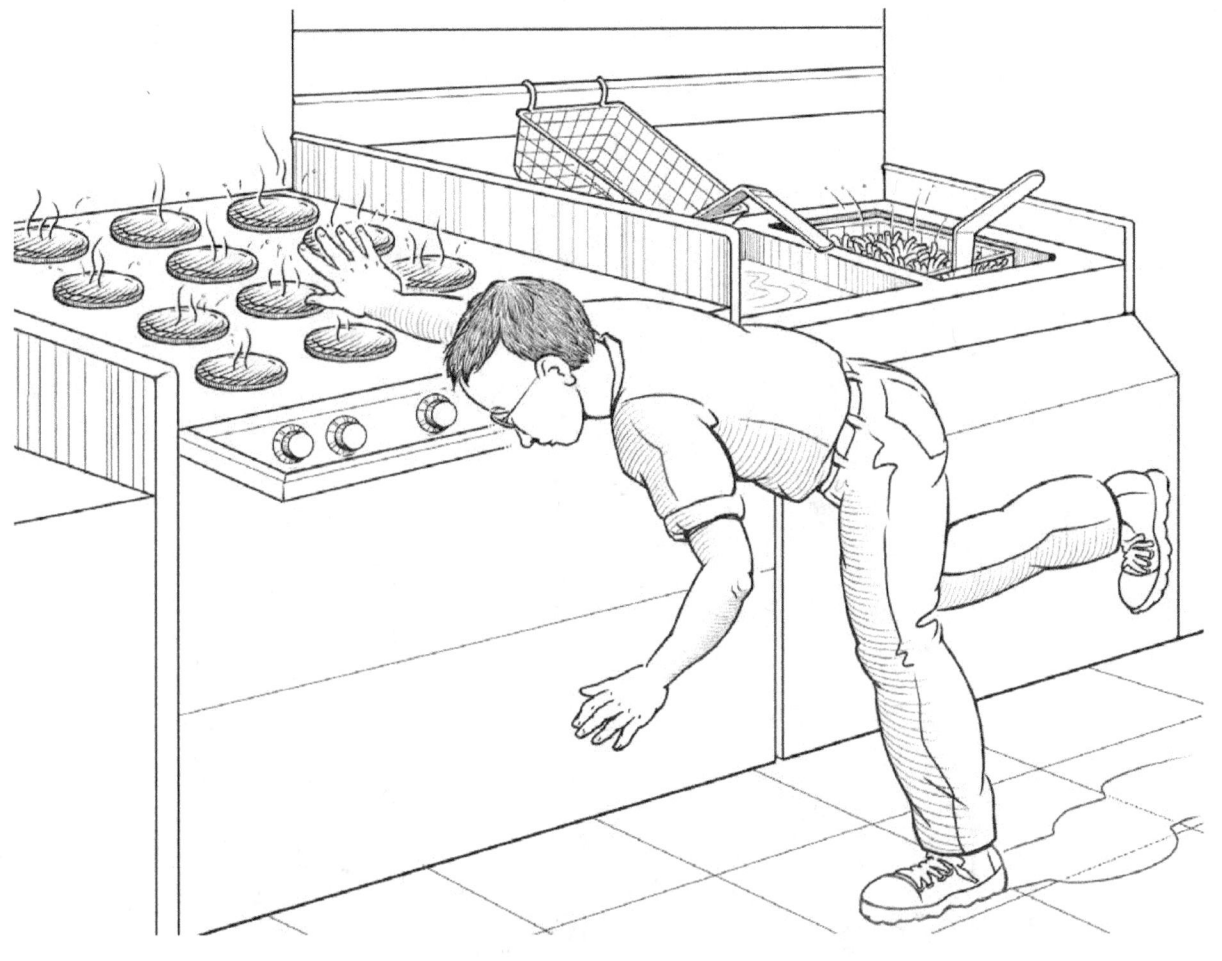

Job: Fast food worker

Injury: Burned hand on grill

Stephen's Story

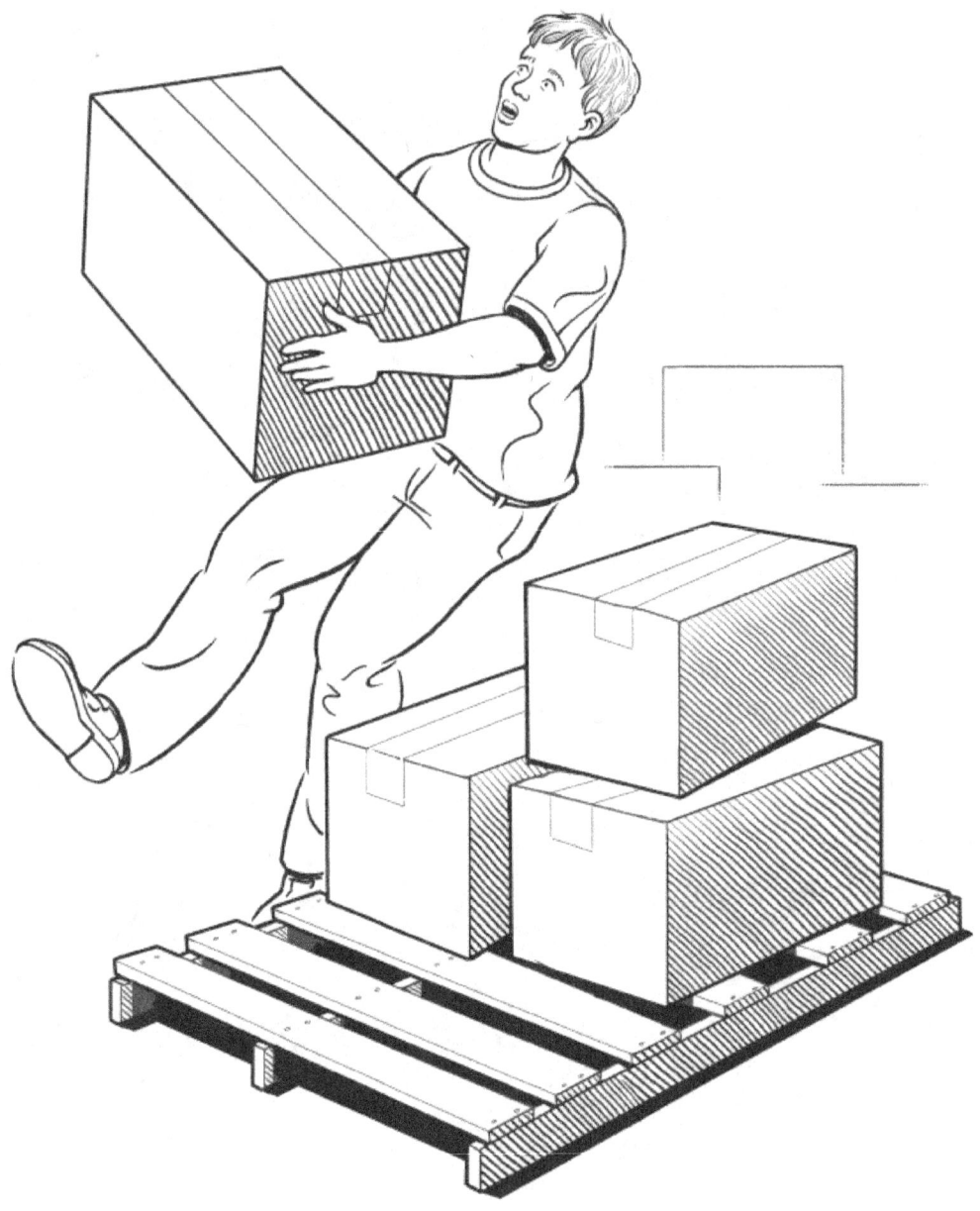

Job: Grocery store clerk

Injury: Hurt back while loading boxes

Terry's Story

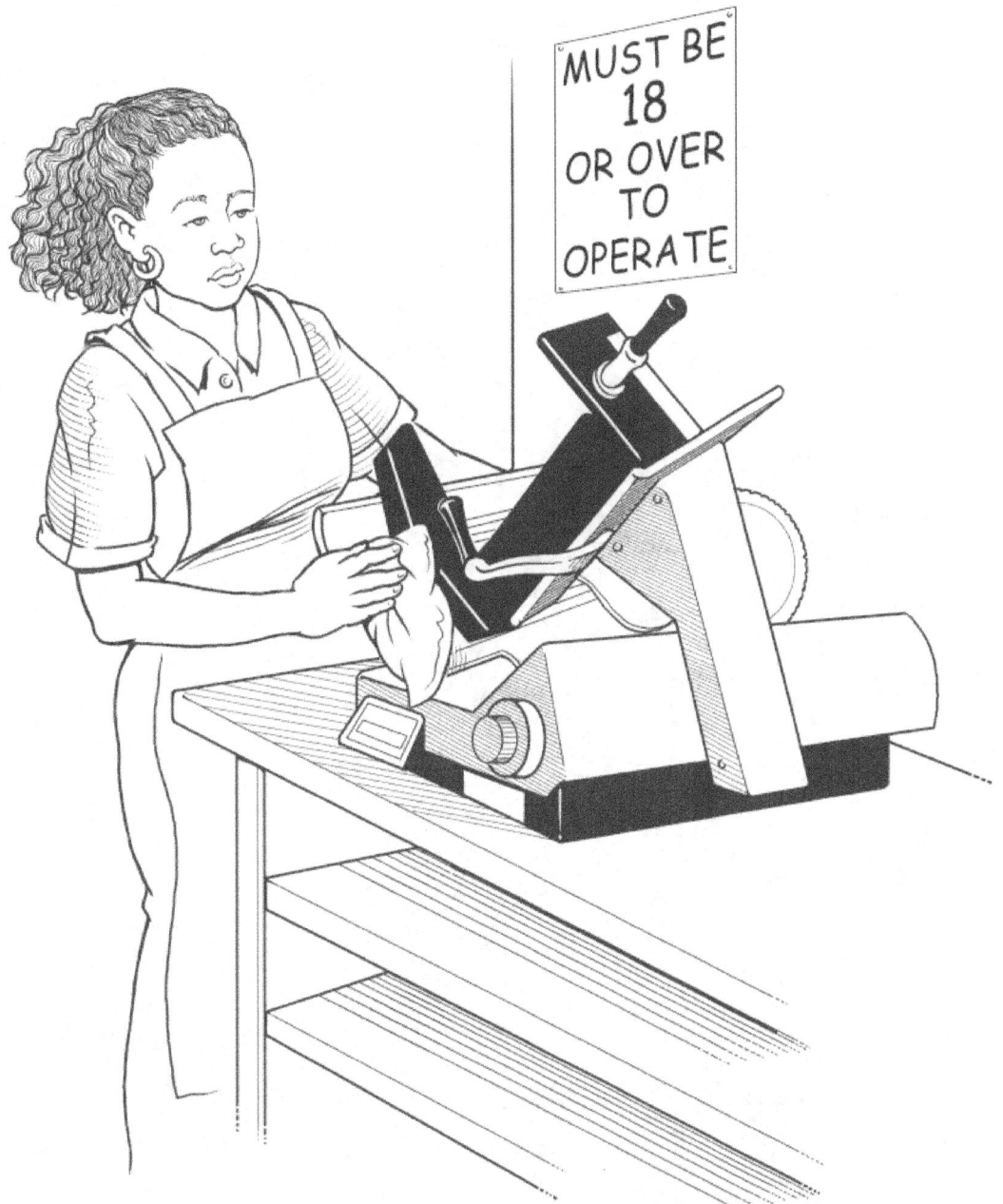

MUST BE
18
OR OVER
TO
OPERATE

Job: Grocery store deli clerk

Injury: Cut finger on meat slicer

Chris' Story

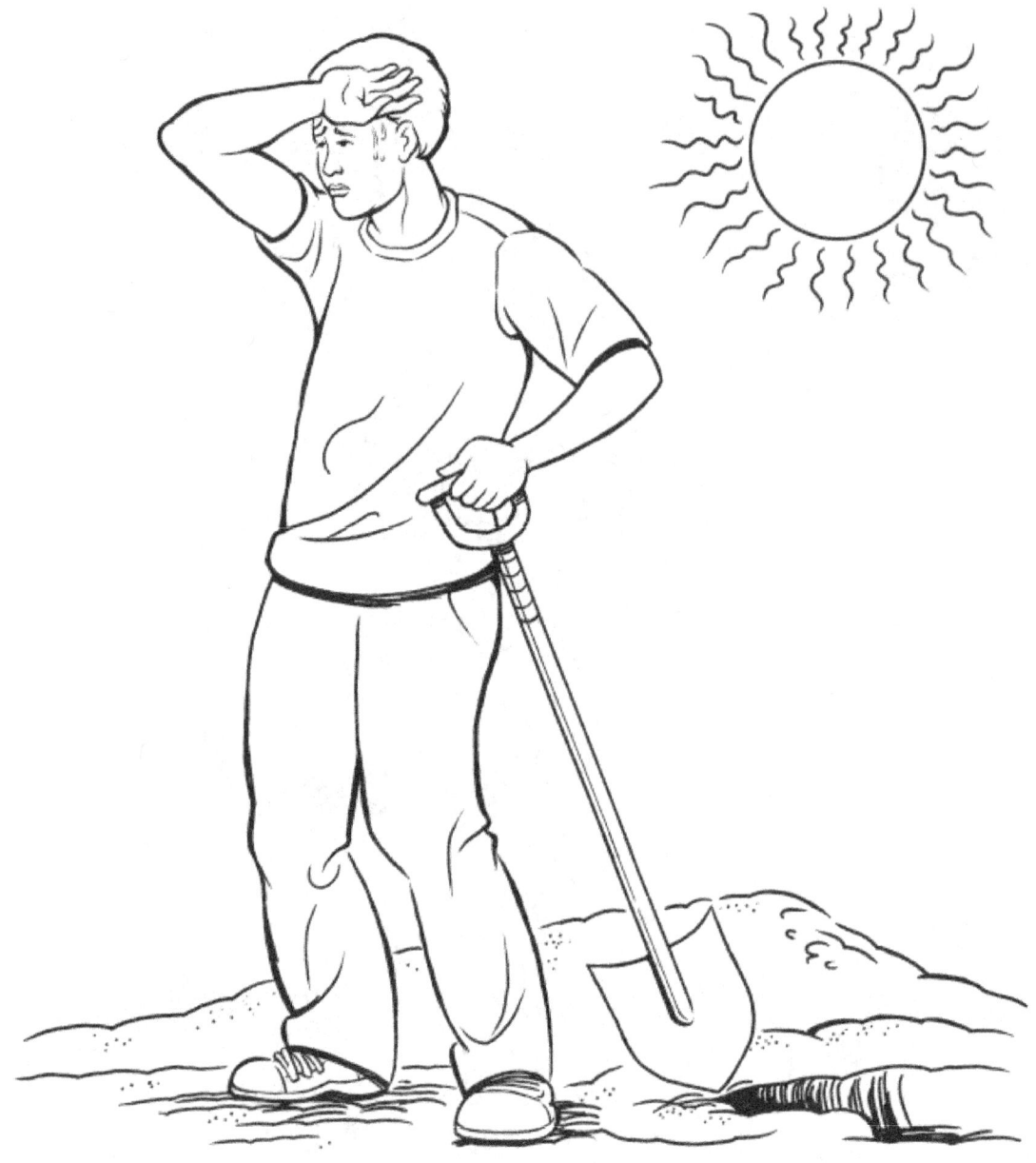

Job: City public works employee

Injury: Fainted due to heat

James' Story

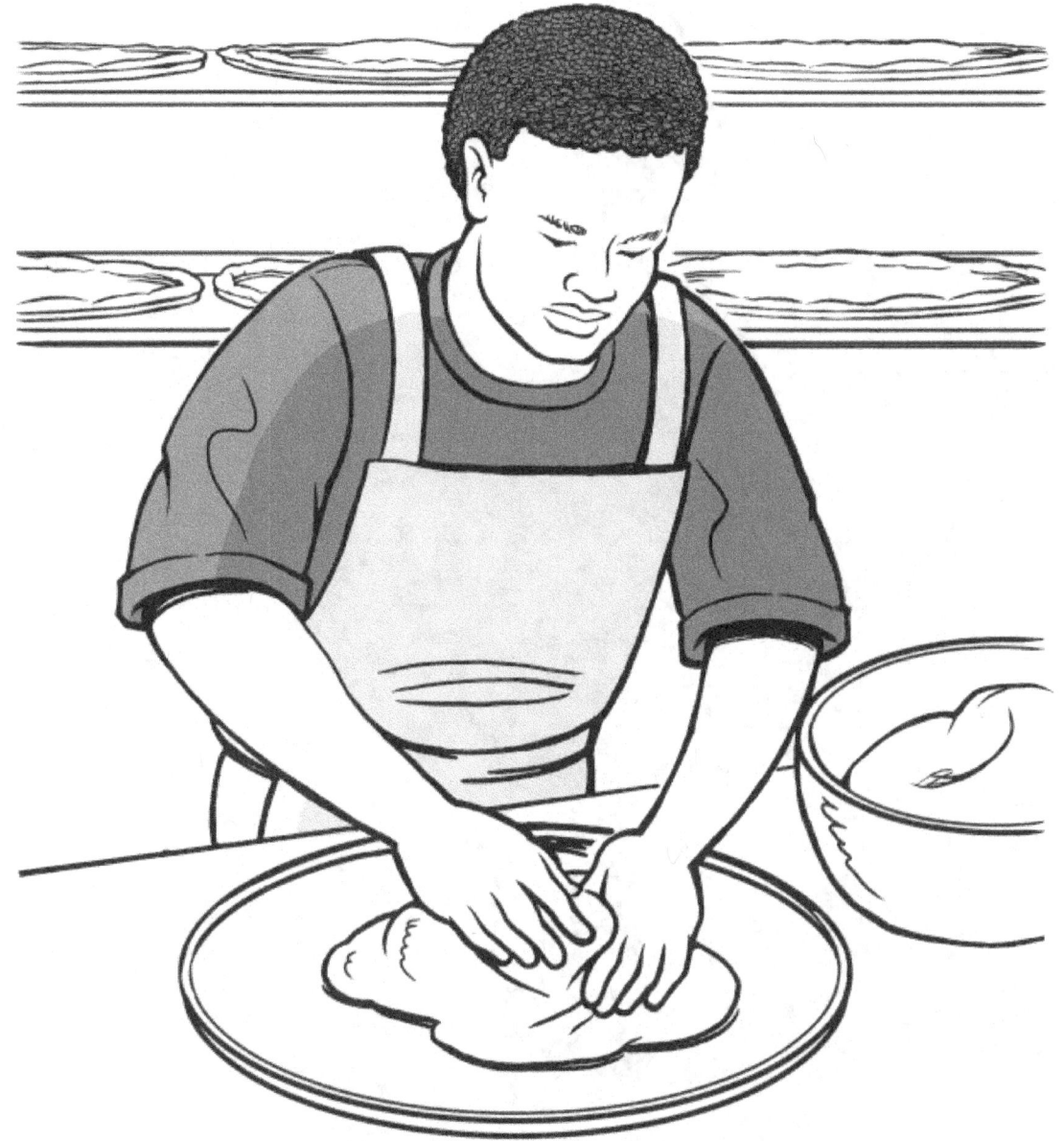

Job: Pizza shop employee

Injury: Repetitive motion injury

Maria's Story

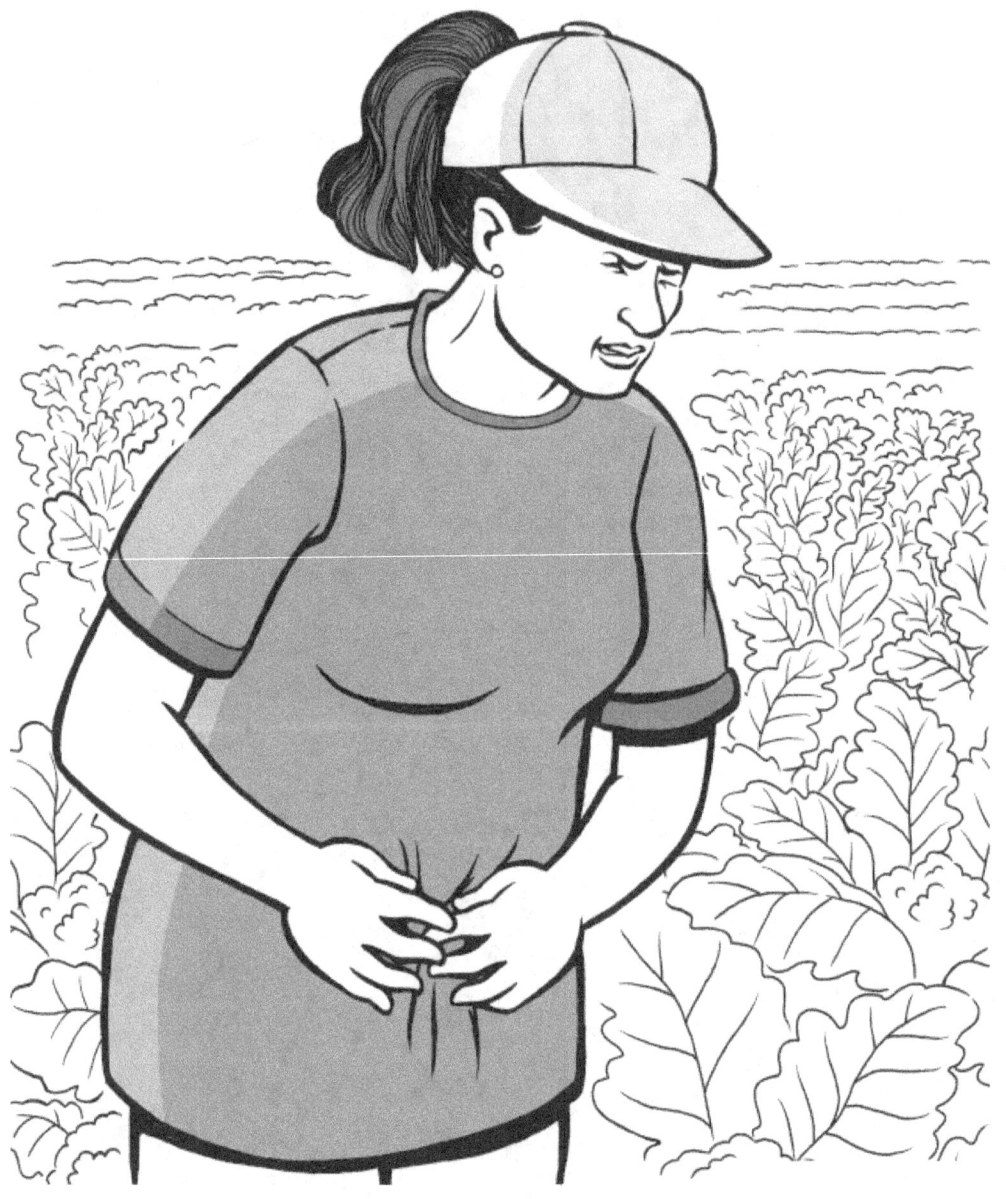

Job: Farmworker

Injury: Pesticide poisoning

Sara's Story

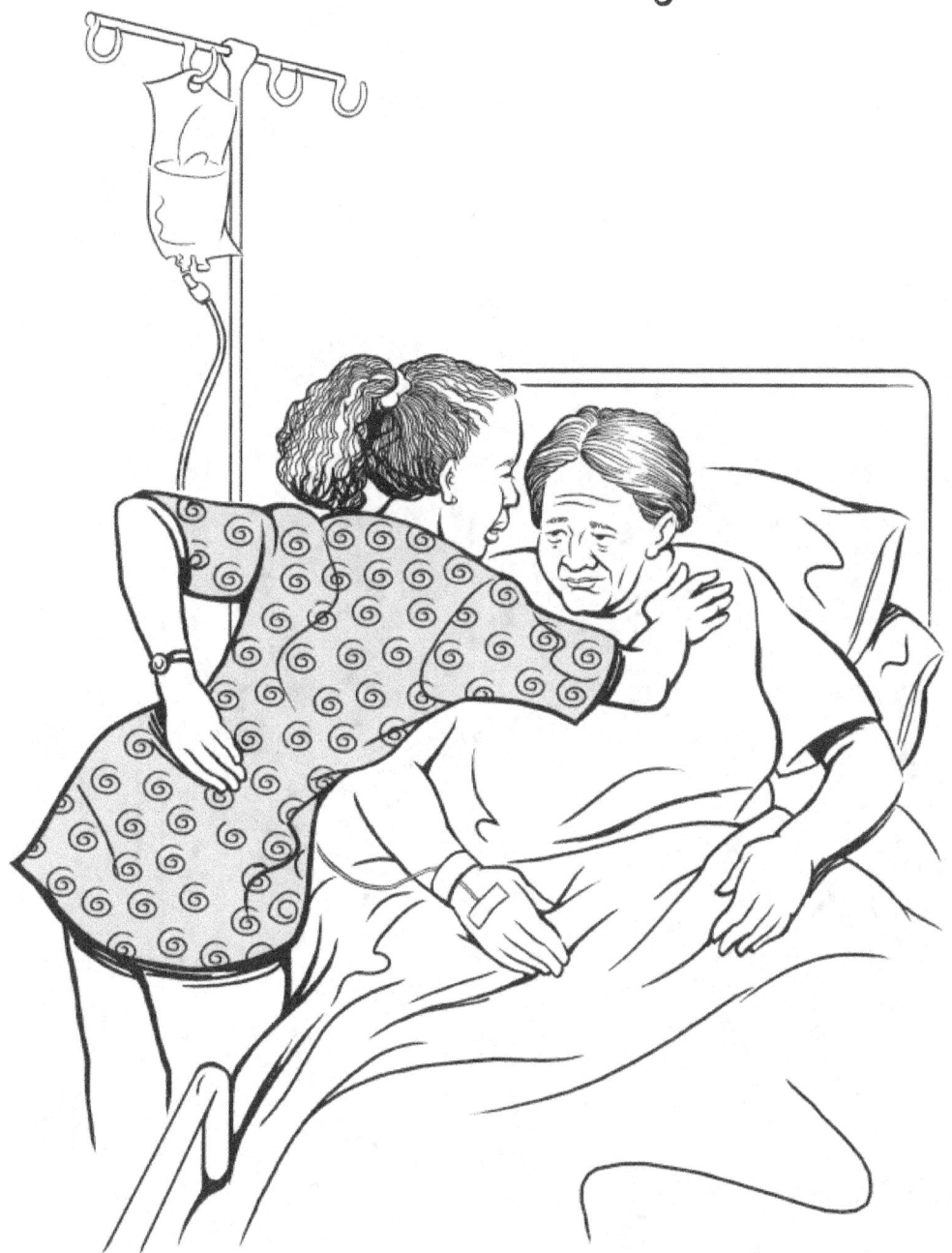

Job: Nursing aide

Injury: Back, neck, and shoulder pain

Brent's Story

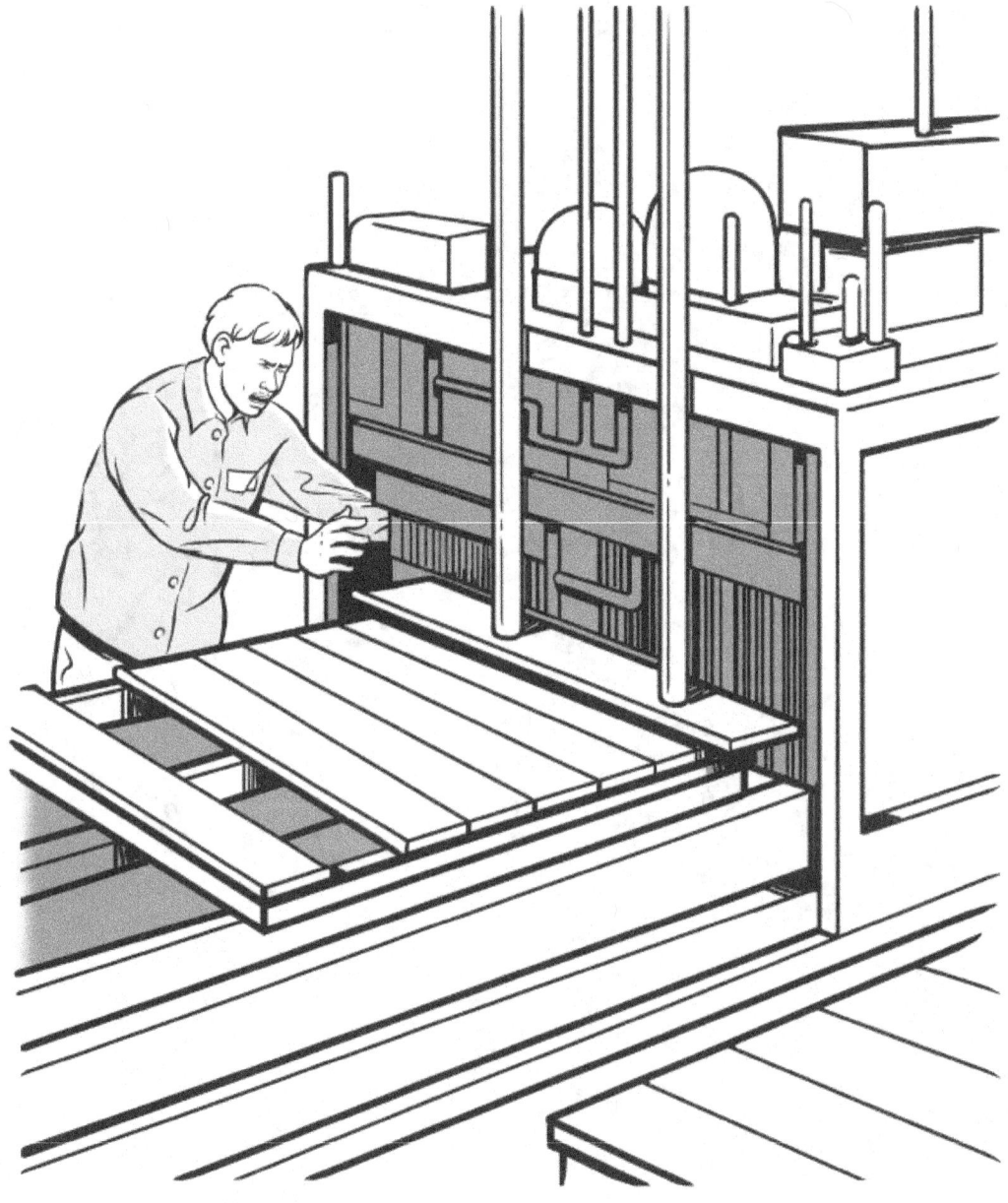

Job: Pallet making

Injury: Amputated arm

Key Points: Making the Job Safer

- OSHA requires employers to provide a safe workplace.

- It's best to get rid of a hazard completely, if possible.

- If your employer can't get rid of the hazard, there are usually many ways to protect you from it.

Key Points: Emergencies at Work

- Every workplace should have an Emergency Action Plan.

- The plan should cover:

  - what to do in different emergencies

  - where shelters and meeting places are

  - evacuation routes

  - emergency equipment and alert systems

  - who's in charge

  - procedures to follow when someone is injured

- The plan should provide for practice drills.

- Workers should be trained on everything in the plan.

Game Board

Rights on the Job	Dangerous Work & Work Permits	Hours for Teens & Working Safely	Job Injuries & Getting Help
$100	$100	$100	$100
$200	$200	$200	$200
$300	$300	$300	$300
$400	$400	$400	$400
$500	$500	$500	$500

Key Points: Know Your Rights

Federal and state labor laws:

- Set a minimum age for some types of dangerous work.

- Protect teens from working too long, too late, or too early.

OSHA says every employer must provide:

- A safe and healthy workplace.

- Safety training on certain hazards, including information on dangerous chemicals.

- Safety equipment.

By law, your employer is not allowed to fire or punish you for reporting a safety problem.

Handling Workplace Safety Problems

- Define the problem.

- Get advice from a parent, teacher, or co-worker.

- Choose your goals. Decide which solution is best.

- Know your rights.

- Decide the best way to talk to the supervisor.

- If necessary, contact an outside agency for help.

Summing Up

- **Know Your Rights.** The factsheet is an important resource. Show it to your friends and parents.

- **Know Your Responsibilities.** It's your responsibility to follow safety rules and report any problems you see.

- **Know Your Employer's Responsibilities.** Your employer must keep the workplace safe and give you safety training.

- **Know How To Solve Problems.** Resources include co-workers, friends, parents, teachers, and government agencies like OSHA, EPA, and federal and state labor law enforcement agencies.

Your Safety IQ Quiz

Work together in your group to answer these questions. Guessing is OK. You won't be graded on your answers. Pick one person in your group to report your answers to the class later.

✔ Check the correct answer.

1. The law says your employer must give you training about health and safety hazards on your job.

   ☐ True   ☐ False   ☐ Don't know

2. The law sets limits on how late you may work on a school night if you are under 16.

   ☐ True   ☐ False   ☐ Don't know

3. If you are 16 years old, you are allowed to drive a car on public streets as part of your job.

   ☐ True   ☐ False   ☐ Don't know

4. If you're injured on the job, your employer must pay for your medical care.

   ☐ True   ☐ False   ☐ Don't know

5. How many teens get seriously injured on the job in the U.S.?

   ☐ One per day   ☐ One per hour   ☐ One every 10 minutes   ☐ Don't know

Find the Hazards: Fast Food

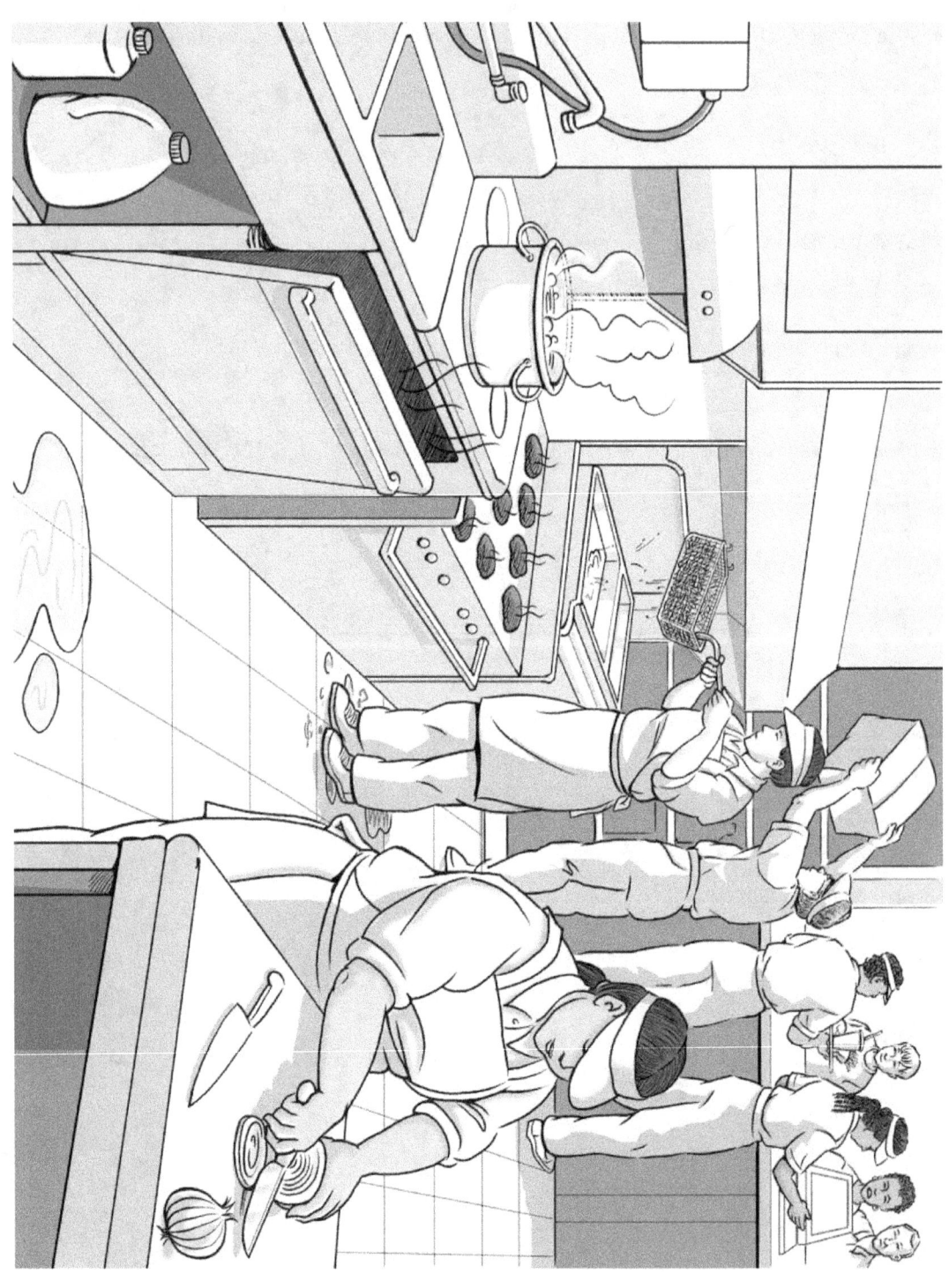

Find the Hazards: Grocery Store

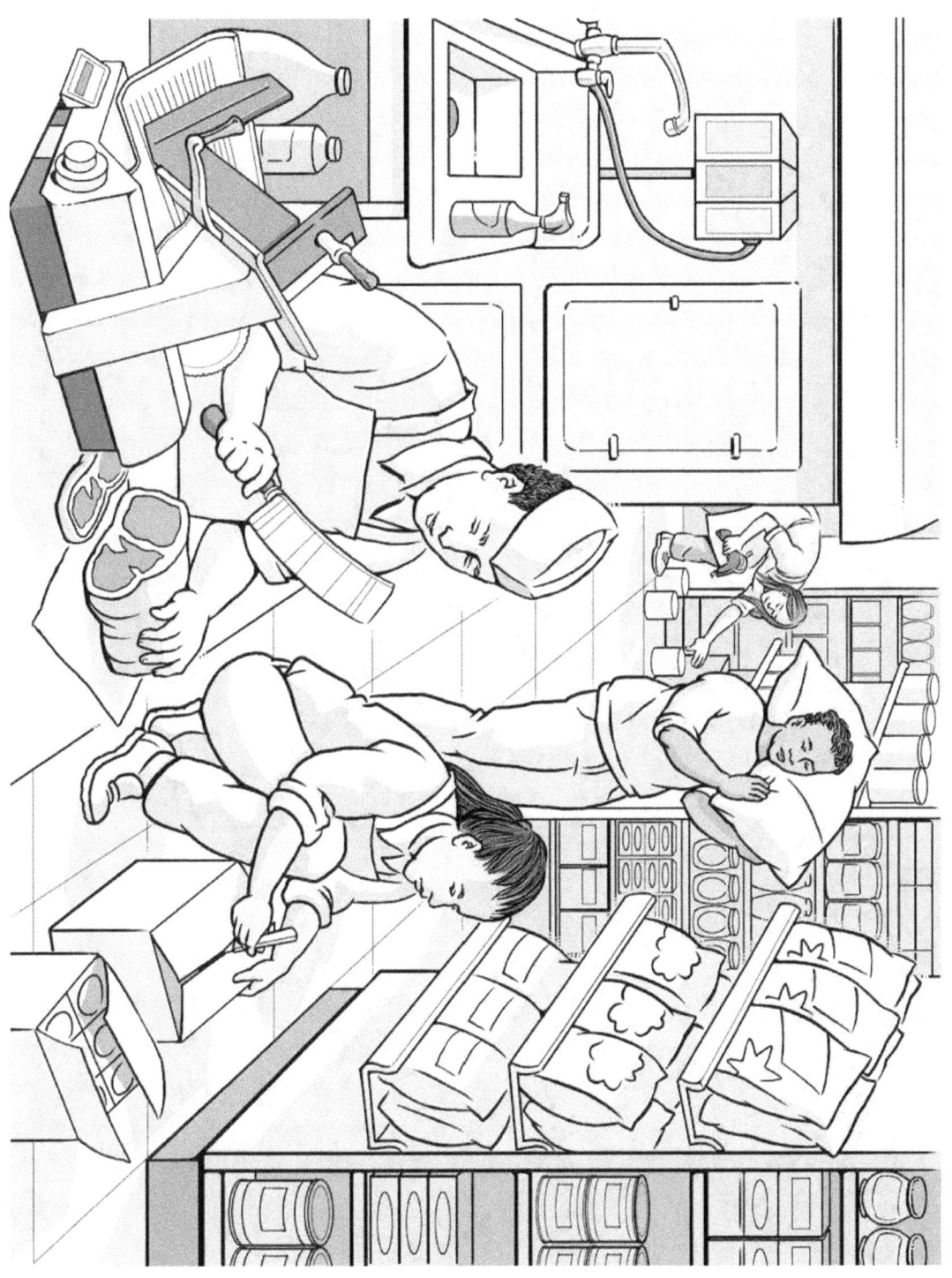

Find the Hazards: Office

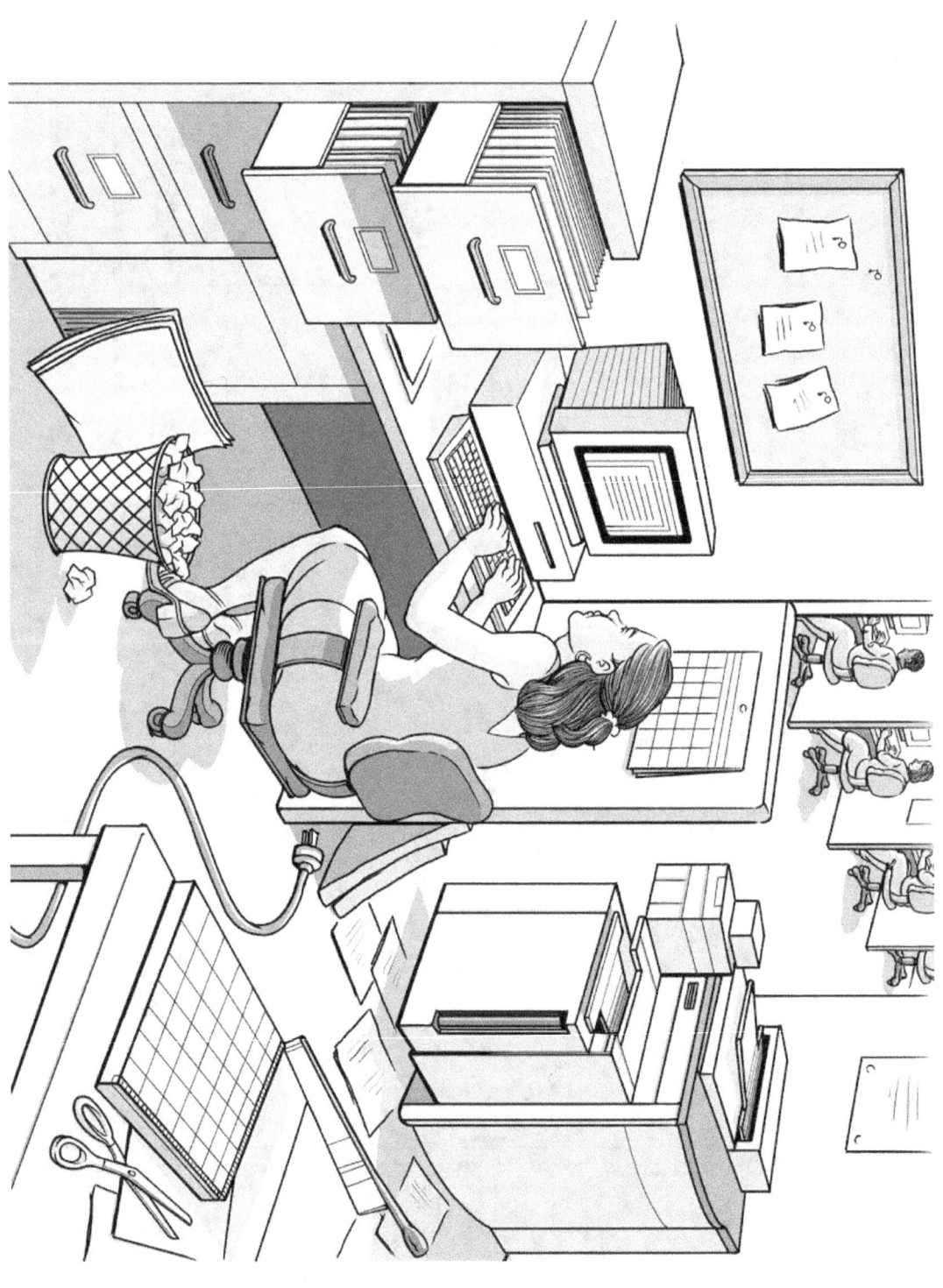

Find the Hazards: Gas Station

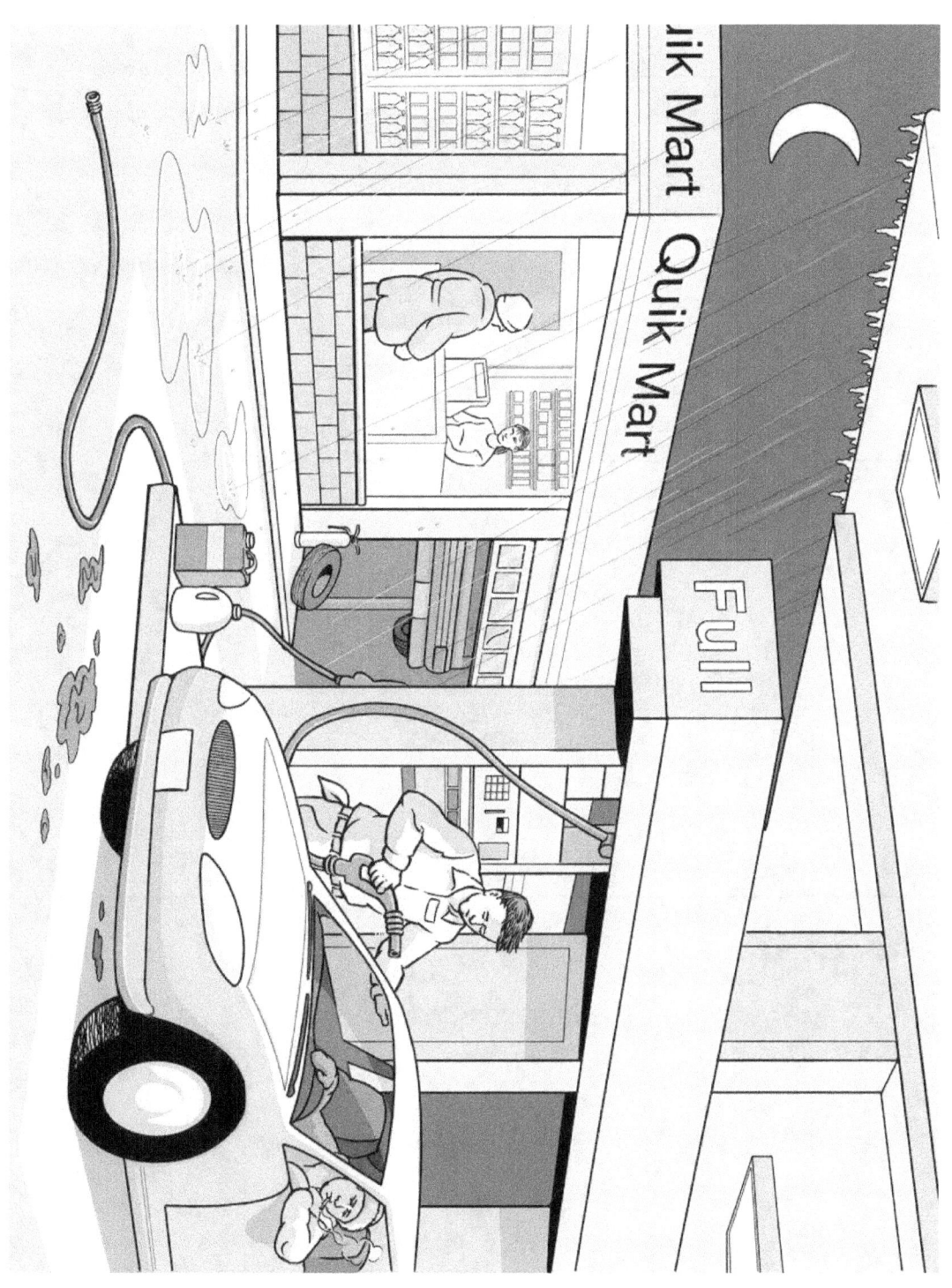

Hunting for Hazards

	Hazard	Possible Harm
Kitchen		

Office

Other Area (_____)

Info Search

A. Worksheet

Your team will be assigned one scenario to research from part C of this handout. Work with your team to answer the questions below. Once all team members have completed their research, discuss and agree on the answers you want to report to the rest of the class. Pick someone in your team to make a brief report.

1. What is the health and safety problem (hazard) in your scenario?

2. What information might you be able to get at the workplace? Where would you get it?

3. Pick three possible sources outside the workplace where you could get information. These must include at least one government agency, and at least one organization or agency that is not part of the government. You can search the internet, or request information by phone. A few suggested resources are listed in part B of this handout. However, you do not need to limit yourself to these. Each team member can get information from a different source, or you can work together. Use these sources to answer the following questions.

   Short-term health effects. How could this hazard affect your body right away?

Information	Source

Long-term health effects. How could this hazard affect your body over time?

Information	Source

Solutions. What are some possible ways to reduce or eliminate workers' exposure to this hazard?

Information	Source

4. What was the most important information you learned, and why was it important?

5. Which information source did your team find most useful, and why?

B. Resources: Where To Get Information

Here are some websites and phone numbers to get factsheets and other information on health and safety hazards.

Government Agencies

New Jersey Occupational Health Services

Website contains "Right To Know—Hazardous Substance Fact Sheets" for over 1500 chemicals.

http://www.state.nj.us/health/eoh/rtkweb/rtkhsfs.htm

NIOSH (National Institute for Occupational Safety and Health)

Conducts research on hazards and has free publications on chemicals, ergonomics, child labor, and other hazards.

www.cdc.gov/niosh/
www.cdc.gov/niosh/topics/youth (Young Worker Safety and Health)

1-800-CDC-INFO (1-800-232-4636)

OSHA (U.S. Occupational Safety and Health Administration)

Develops and enforces federal regulations and standards. Offers free publications and a video library.

www.osha.gov/SLTC/

(800) 321-OSHA

Other Organizations

AFL-CIO Safety and Health on the Job

Basic health and safety information, including an alphabetical listing of direct links to fact sheets developed by unions and OSHA. Some are available in Spanish.

http://www.aflcio.org/issues/safety/tools/infofs.cfm

Labor Occupational Health Program (LOHP), University of California, Berkeley

Trains workers, unions, joint labor-management committees, and others on health and safety. Sells publications and videos. Offers assistance and referrals on young workers, workplace violence, hazardous waste, ergonomics, and more.

www.lohp.org

(510) 642-5507

NYCOSH (New York Committee for Occupational Safety and Health)

Website has internet links and resources on health and safety by industry and topic, as well as basic information on health and safety rights on the job.

www.nycosh.org/

Vermont SIRI (Safety Information Resources Inc.)

Website contains links to many health and safety resources. Specializes in Material Safety Data Sheets.

www.siri.org

C. Scenarios

Scenario A: Big Box Foods

Kevin works in a warehouse. He's seventeen years old. One day, when he was loading 40-pound boxes onto a wooden pallet, he suddenly felt a sharp pain in his lower back. He had to stay out of work for a week to recover, and his back still hurts sometimes. He is worried about re-injuring his back, and tries to be careful, but he wants to find out more about safe lifting and other ways to prevent back injuries.

Scenario B: Brian's Computer Station

Brian has been working for six months as an administrative assistant in a large office. He is the newest employee in the office, and seems to have all the hand-me-down equipment. His keyboard and mouse sit right on his desktop, along with his computer monitor. The lever to adjust the height of his chair doesn't work any more. He works at his computer most of the day. He knows at least one person in the office who wears braces on her wrists because they are tender and painful, and who can no longer do a lot of things at home because her grip is so weak. Brian doesn't want to develop any problems like that, and wants to find out what he can do.

Scenario C: Dangerous Paint Stripper

Jessica has a summer job working for the city parks program. She has been using a cleaner called "Graffiti Gone" to remove graffiti from the bathrooms. She has to take a lot of breaks, because the chemical makes her throat burn. It also makes her feel dizzy sometimes, especially when the bathrooms don't have very many windows. On the label, she sees that the cleaner has methylene chloride in it. She feels like she's managing to get the work done, but she is worried about feeling dizzy. She wants to find out more about this chemical, what harm it can cause, and whether there are safer ways to do this work.

Scenario D: Noise at Work

Ediberto is 18 years old, and has been working for a company that manufactures prefabricated homes for about a year. He spends a lot of the work day using a power saw. His ears usually ring for awhile in the evening, but it seems to clear up by the morning. He is a little worried about whether it's damaging his hearing, but it's not that different than how his ears feel after a rock concert. He wants to find some information on how much noise is bad for you, and what he can do.

Scenario E: Needles in the Laundry Stack

Simone works as an aide in a nursing home. Her best friend's cousin Julia works in the laundry department. Simone has heard Julia complain about the medical staff, because used hypodermic needles sometimes show up in the dirty laundry. Simone is worried about Julia, but also doesn't think the medical staff could be that careless. She wants more information on what can be done.

Scenario F: Stop and Shop

Sarah works in a convenience store. She and the other employees take turns working the closing shift. It makes her nervous to be at the store by herself late at night, but she knows if she refuses the closing shifts, the owner will just look for someone else for the job. She carries mace in her purse, and the owner has told her to give up the cash in the cash register if she is ever faced with a robber, but she wants to find out what else can be done so she will feel safe.

Disaster Blaster Game Board

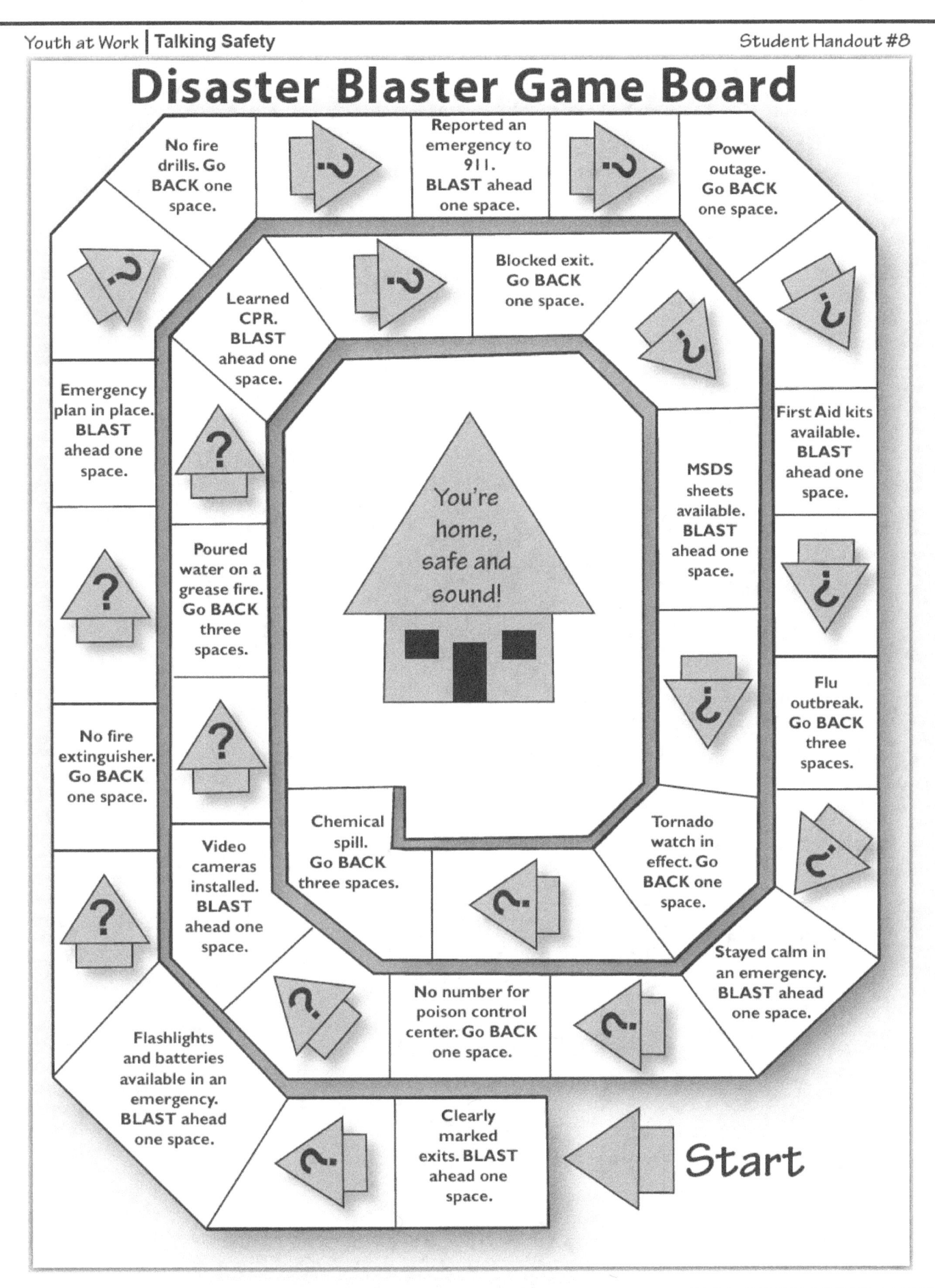

No fire drills. Go **BACK** one space.

Reported an emergency to 911. **BLAST** ahead one space.

Power outage. **Go BACK** one space.

Blocked exit. **Go BACK** one space.

Learned CPR. **BLAST** ahead one space.

Emergency plan in place. **BLAST** ahead one space.

First Aid kits available. **BLAST** ahead one space.

You're home, safe and sound!

MSDS sheets available. **BLAST** ahead one space.

Poured water on a grease fire. **Go BACK** three spaces.

Flu outbreak. **Go BACK** three spaces.

No fire extinguisher. **Go BACK** one space.

Video cameras installed. **BLAST** ahead one space.

Chemical spill. **Go BACK** three spaces.

Tornado watch in effect. Go **BACK** one space.

Stayed calm in an emergency. **BLAST** ahead one space.

No number for poison control center. Go **BACK** one space.

Flashlights and batteries available in an emergency. **BLAST** ahead one space.

Clearly marked exits. **BLAST** ahead one space.

Start

Disaster Blaster Game Cards

Q. If you are inside a building and begin to feel the shaking of an earthquake, what should you do?

A. Get under something heavy or sturdy like a desk or doorframe.

Q. If you are in a building and hear a tornado warning, what should you do?

A. Go to the lowest level of the building; the basement, a storm shelter, or an interior room without windows.

Q. If you smell smoke and suspect a fire burning somewhere in the building, what should you do?

A. Alert others. Pull fire alarm if available. Shut door and get out of the building. Call 911 from outside.

Q. If someone comes into your workplace with a gun, what should you do?

A. Cooperate fully with the gunman's instructions, Don't try to be a hero.

Q. If an unknown chemical spills in your workplace, what should you do?

A. Leave it alone and get your supervisor.

Q. How many exit routes must a workplace have?

A. Enough to allow for safe evacuation of all employees (and customers) but at least two exits.

Q. True or False? If you are caught in a fire you should stay close to the ground.

A. True.

Q. What are the steps for using a fire extinguisher?

A. P-A-S-S:
Pull the pin;
Aim the nozzle;
Squeeze the trigger;
Sweep extinguisher back and forth over the fire.

Q. What phone number should you call to report an emergency?

A. 911.

Q. What should you do for a severe cut?

A. Apply pressure to the wound and, if there are no broken bones, elevate the wound above the heart. Seek medical help.

Q. What should you do for a very serious second or third degree heat burn?

A. Call 911. Don't remove clothing if stuck to the burned area.

Q. What should be used to put out a grease fire on a stove?

A. A pan lid or baking soda. *Never* water or flour.

Q. What should you do if you are in a building and the power goes out?

A. Stay calm. If appropriate to leave, look for lighted exit signs. Otherwise, stay in place and check with your supervisor.

Q. On the way home from work late one night, your car breaks down on an isolated road. What do you do?

A. Turn on hazard lights. Lock doors, stay in car. Call for help, wait for assistance. Or put sign up asking passers- by to call 911. Do not open car to strangers.

Q. You are working on a construction site and a co-worker enters a trench and passes out. What do you do?

A. Tell a supervisor. Don't go after him; you may become a second victim. Call 911.

Q. A co-worker slips on a wet floor, hits his head, and loses consciousness. What do you do?

A. Don't move him. Call 911. Check breathing and heartbeat. Give CPR if you can. Cover and keep him warm.

Q. If a co-worker falls off a ladder and injures his back, what should you do?

A. Don't move him (this can cause more damage). Call 911 for help.

Q. If your clothes catch on fire, what should you do?

A. Stop, drop, and roll; or smother the flames with a blanket. Never run.

Q. Name at least one factor that increases your risk of being robbed at work?

A. Working alone; working at night; access to money.

Q. What letters are on the type of fire extinguisher that can be used in any kind of fire?

A. A–B–C.
(A) Trash, wood, paper;
(B) Liquids, gasses, solvents;
(C) Electrical equipment.

Q. What is the name of the sheets that provide information about chemical products?

A. Material Safety Data Sheets—MSDSs.

Q. What is at least one item that should be included in an emergency kit?

A. Water; flashlight and batteries; first aid supplies.

Q. What does the skull and crossbones symbol mean?

A. Poison.

Q. If a chemical gets into your eye, what should you do?

A. Flush it with water for at least 15 minutes.

Q. Name one security measure that can reduce workplace violence in a retail store?

A. Good lighting; a panic button or other communication device; a security guard; a video camera.

Q. How do you prevent the spread of flu viruses?

A. Cover nose / mouth with a tissue when coughing / sneezing. Wash hands, don't touch eyes, nose, or mouth. Stay home.

Q. What two common cleaning products should you never mix, because they make a gas that can kill you?

A. Ammonia and bleach (the mixture releases chlorine gas, which can be deadly).

Q. What's the difference between a weather watch and a weather warning?

A. *Watch*: Severe weather possible during the next few hours. *Warning*: Severe weather observed or expected soon.

Q. If you are driving to work and see the funnel shape of a tornado approaching, what should you do?

A. Get out of the car and lie down in a low place.

Q. If you are working outside when a lightning storm starts and you can't get to shelter, what should you do?

A. Crouch low to the ground, sit on the balls of your feet, stay away from trees and metal objects.

Q. What do you do if you come in contact with a substance, but don't know whether or not it is toxic?

A. Call the National Poison Control Center: 1-800-222-1222.

Q. What can you use to melt ice on the sidewalks in the winter?

A. Rock salt

Q. Name at least two things that should be in an Emergency Action Plan.

A. Name of person who is in charge; escape routes; training; drills; alarm systems; meeting place.

Q. What does CPR stand for and what is it?

A. Cardiopulmonary Resuscitation. CPR is a combination of rescue breathing and chest compressions for a victim whose heart has stopped beating.

Q. Is it safe to use a cell phone or cordless phone during a storm?

A. Yes. These are safe to use because there is no direct path between you and the lightning. Use a corded telephone *only* in an emergency.

Q. If a co-worker suffers from heat exhaustion, what should you do?

A. Get the person out of the sun. Give her cool water. Lay the person down and elevate her feet. Call 911.

Emergencies in the News

In your small group, read your assigned news story, then answer the three questions on the other side.

Story A: Grease Fire in Restaurant Burns Employee

A fire erupted at Sunny's Family Restaurant Tuesday night, critically injuring an employee and causing $100,000 worth of damage to the building. The fire was caused when a frying pan, filled with oil heating up on the stove, was left unattended. The fire rapidly spread to dish towels hanging nearby. An employee discovered the scene and attempted to put out the fire by pouring water on the stove, causing the burning grease to splatter all over his face, arms, and chest. A co-worker, hearing the commotion, called 911 and yelled for everyone to leave the restaurant immediately. The fire department arrived, extinguished the fire, and attended to the burned employee. The victim was taken to Mercy Hospital and is reported to be in serious but stable condition.

Story B: Robber Threatens Young Employee With Gun

A 16-year-old employee of a local convenience store was held up at gunpoint late Thursday night by a masked man demanding money. The employee was working alone and in the process of closing the store for the evening. The employee later reported to police that, after emptying the cash register, the robber tied him up and then left with the money. Although the young employee was shaken up by the incident, he was not physically injured. The name of the young employee is being withheld because of his age.

Story C: Parents Praise Quick Action of Local Teen

Parents Charlene Cook and Kelly Nelson, who have children attending the Happy Go Lucky Day Care Center, called the Daily Times this week to praise the quick action of 17-year-old Tamara Thompson, one of Happy Go Lucky's star employees. Tamara noticed that an entire container of bleach had spilled near the janitor's closet and was giving off fumes in one of the nearby classrooms. Knowing that some of the children have asthma, Tamara walked the children to another teacher's classroom so they wouldn't be exposed. She then rushed back with paper towels to clean up the spill. Unfortunately, Tamara herself suffered breathing problems after cleaning up the bleach and had to be taken to the emergency room to be checked. She is currently at home recovering but plans to return to work when she feels better.

Story D: Young Construction Worker Falls From Ladder

An 18-year-old house painter, who was painting the second story of a house, fell off his ladder yesterday, breaking both legs. He also suffered severe cuts when he caught his arm on a metal fence during the fall. Co-workers rushed to assist him and called for an ambulance. Local EMTs reported that the co-workers carried the fallen employee to the front lawn and then applied pressure to the open wound to stop the bleeding.

Story E: 6.1 Earthquake Shakes Local High Rise Office Building

Office workers at R&D Business Solutions huddled under desks and doorways as a 6.1 earthquake shook their building. Once the tremors subsided, they followed lighted exit signs to the stairwell. They made it down ten flights of stairs and outside to the street. Gladys Royce, of Washington Township, whose son, Jason, is an employee of the company, complained that her son, who has Down Syndrome, was left alone to figure out what to do during and after the earthquake. The employees and supervisors had no idea Jason had remained on the 11th floor. The company pledges to take another look at its Emergency Action Plan and make sure the plan protects and prepares all their employees, including those who may need extra assistance.

Story F: Tornado Breaks Windows at Local Department Store

A tornado blew through town yesterday, causing major power outages and damage to several buildings, including blowing out most of the windows in Johnson's Department Store on East 8th Street. As glass went flying, employees reportedly herded customers into the center section of each floor in the three-story building. Customer Tom Wilson expressed appreciation for the assistance employees provided in getting everyone away from the windows.

Questions

1. What went right in this situation?

2. What went wrong in this situation?

3. What steps should be taken in this workplace to make sure employees are better protected and prepared the next time?

Emergency Action Plans

Planning ahead can reduce the effects of an emergency on workers, the workplace property, and the surrounding community. In preparing an Emergency Action Plan, an employer can figure out what protections are needed and what procedures should be followed in an emergency. All workplaces should have an Emergency Action Plan.

An Emergency Action Plan should be in writing. It should state who is responsible for coordinating emergency response; where chemicals are stored and where Material Safety Data Sheets (MSDSs) for these chemicals are kept; and how critical operations will be maintained during and after an emergency (if necessary). The plan should also list measures that will be taken to protect employees (including those with physical disabilities).

Training and drills

There should be training and regular practice drills so everyone knows what to do during different kinds of emergencies. Workers should be trained so they understand their responsibilities during an emergency; the alarm system and "all clear" announcements; where to gather during an emergency; how to report an emergency; what to do if there is a chemical spill; and when and how to use emergency equipment.

Alarm systems

These must be seen, heard, and understood by all employees.

Shelters and evacuation

The plan should designate inside shelters, exits, evacuation routes and procedures, and outside meeting places. Shelters inside the building should be identified if tornadoes or hurricanes are a possibility. Exits and evacuation routes should be checked periodically to be sure they are not blocked. Exits should be of sufficient number, width, and location that workers can rapidly evacuate. An outside meeting place should be designated so employees can be counted after evacuation.

Emergency lighting

Exit routes should have emergency lighting in all areas where work is performed after daylight hours.

Emergency equipment

The plan should provide for installation and testing of appropriate emergency equipment such as building sprinkler systems, fire extinguishers, eyewash systems, and safety showers if chemicals are used.

Procedures to follow when someone is injured

First aid kits should be provided, as well as trained personnel to use them. Employees should know who is trained in first aid or CPR, and where to get medical attention if needed.

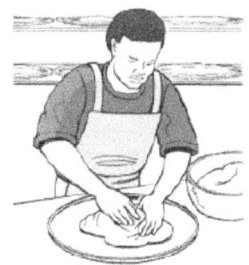

Are You a Working Teen in
North Carolina?

Protect Your Health!
Know Your Rights!

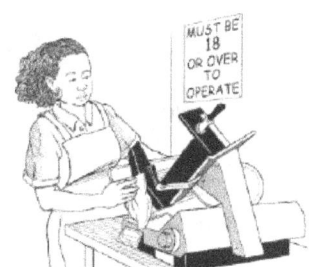

Could I get hurt or sick on the job?

- 18-year-old Sylvia caught her hand in an electric cabbage shredder at a fast food restaurant. Her hand is permanently disfigured and she'll never have full use of it again.

- 17-year-old Joe lost his life while working as a construction helper. An electric shock killed him when he climbed a metal ladder to hand an electric drill to another worker.

- 16-year-old Donna was assaulted and robbed at gunpoint at a sandwich shop. She was working alone after 11 p.m.

Every year in the United States, 158,000 teens under age 18 are injured in the workplace. Approximately 53,000 young people seek emergency room treatment for their injuries. On average, 48 teens die each year from work-related injuries.

Why do teens get sick or hurt on the job? Injuries to young workers are usually due to unsafe equipment or a hazardous environment, stressful conditions, or working too fast to meet a deadline. As a young worker, you are more likely to be injured on jobs that the law does not allow you to do.

What hazards should I watch out for?

Type of work	Examples of hazards
Food Service	Slippery floors Hot cooking equipment Sharp objects
Retail/Sales	Violent crimes Harassment Heavy lifting
Office/Clerical	Stress Harassment Poor computer work station design
Janitor/Clean-up	Toxic chemicals in cleaning products Blood on discarded needles
Farm/Agricultural	Unsafe machinery Chemicals in pesticides Slippery surfaces and confined spaces

What are my rights on the job?

By law, your employer must provide:

- A safe and healthful workplace.

- Training on chemicals and other health and safety hazards.

- Protective clothing and equipment.

- (At least) the federal minimum wage of $7.25 per hour. Some jobs are exempt from minimum wage laws. **For more details, see www.dol.gov/whd/minwage/america.htm.**

- Workers' compensation benefits if you are hurt on the job. These include:

  - ➤ Medical care for your injury, whether or not you miss time from work.

  - ➤ Payments if you lose wages for more than seven days.

  - ➤ Other benefits if you become permanently disabled.

You also have a right to:

- Report safety problems to OSHA.

- Work free of discrimination and harassment because of your race, color, religion, sex (including pregnancy), national origin, disability, age (age 40 or older), or sexual orientation.

  - ➤ Examples of workplace harassment include: Lewd jokes, racial or ethnic slurs, pressure for sexual favors, unwelcome comments about religion, or offensive pictures or graffiti.

- Report job discrimination without being punished or treated differently by your employer.

- Request reasonable workplace accommodations for religious beliefs or a medical condition.

- Refuse to work if the job is immediately dangerous to your life or health.

- Join or organize a union.

  - ➤ You have a right to engage in group activities to try to improve working conditions, wages, and benefits.

  - ➤ You have a right to talk about your wages with your co-workers.

Is it ok to do any kind of work?

NO! Certain laws protect teens from doing dangerous work.

In North Carolina, no worker under age 18 may:

- Drive a motor vehicle on public streets as part of the job (17-year-olds may drive in very limited circumstances).

- Drive a forklift or other heavy equipment.

- Use powered equipment like a circular saw, box crusher, meat slicer, or bakery machine.

- Work in wrecking, demolition, excavation, or roofing.

- Work in logging or a sawmill.

- Handle, serve, or sell alcohol.

- Work where there is exposure to radiation.

Also, **no one 14 or 15 years old may:**

- Do any baking activities.

- Cook (except with electric or gas grills that do not involve cooking over an open flame and with deep fat fryers that automatically lower and raise the baskets).
- Work in dry cleaning or a commercial laundry.
- Do building, construction, or manufacturing work.
- Load or unload a truck, railroad car, or conveyor.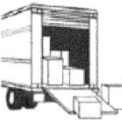
- Work on a ladder or scaffold.

Are there other things I can't do?

YES! There are other restrictions on the type of work you can and cannot do. **Age 14** is the minimum for most employment, except for informal jobs like babysitting or yard work. Check with your state labor department, school counselor, or job placement coordinator to make sure the job you are doing is allowed.

Do I need a work permit?

YES! If you are under 18 and plan to work, you must fill out a youth employment certificate, which is online at: www.nclabor.com/wh/youth_instructions.htm

Also, if you are under age 18 your employer must have on file a copy of your "proof of age" (such as a birth certificate, driver's license, or work permit).

What are my safety responsibilities on the job?

To work safely you should:

- Follow all safety rules and instructions; use safety equipment and protective clothing when needed.
- Look out for co-workers.

- Keep work areas clean and neat.
- Know what to do in an emergency.
- Report any health and safety hazard to your supervisor.
- Ask questions if you don't understand.

You have a right to speak up!

By law, your employer cannot fire or punish you for reporting a workplace problem or injury, or for claiming workers' compensation.

Should I work this late or this long?

Child labor laws protect teens from working too long, too late, or too early.

The table below shows the hours North Carolina teens may work. (Some school districts may have more restrictive regulations. Also, there are some exceptions for teens in work experience education programs).

Work Hours for North Carolina Teens		
	Ages 14 and 15	**Ages 16 and 17**
Work hours	7am–7pm, from Labor Day to June 1 When attendance at school is not required 7am–9pm, from June 1 to Labor Day	5am–11pm when there is school the next day*
Maximum hours when school is in session	18 hours a week, but not more than: 3 hours a day on school days 8 hours a day Saturday to Sunday, and holidays	No limitations
Maximum hours when school is *not* in session	40 hours a week 8 hours a day	No limitations

*Hours restrictions may be waived with written parental consent and written consent from the school principal or designee.

What if I get hurt on the job?

Tell your supervisor right away. If you're under 18, tell your parents or guardians, too. Get emergency medical treatment if needed. Request a **claim form** from your employer, if he/she does not immediately provide one. Fill it out and return it to your employer. This helps ensure that you receive workers' compensation benefits.

Workers' Compensation:

Did You Know?

- You can receive benefits:
  - ➢ Even if you are under 18.
  - ➢ Even if you are a temporary or part-time worker (in most cases).
- You receive benefits no matter who was at fault for your job injury.
- You don't have to be a legal resident of the U.S. to receive benefits.
- You can't sue your employer for a job injury (in most cases).

What if I have a safety problem?

- Talk to your supervisor, parents, teachers, job training representative, or union representative (if any) about the problem.
- Contact NIOSH (National Institute for Occupational Safety and Health) for general safety information.

  (1–800) CDC–INFO (232–4636)
  www.cdc.gov/niosh

- Call the National Young Worker Safety Resource Center for health and safety information and advice. Many materials are available in Spanish.

  (510) 643–2424
  www.youngworkers.org

- Contact one of the following agencies necessary:

To make a health or safety complaint:

- OSHA (Occupational Safety and Health Administration)

  (800) 321–OSHA (6742)
  www.osha.gov

- North Carolina Occupational Safety and Health Division (OSHNC)

  (800) NC-LABOR (625-2267)
  www.nclabor.com/osha/osh.htm

To make a complaint about wages or work hours:

- North Carolina Wage & Hour Bureau

  (800) NC-LABOR (625-2267)
  www.nclabor.com/wh/wh.htm

- U.S. Department of Labor

  (866) 487–9243
  www.dol.gov/whd/

To make a complaint about sexual harassment or discrimination:

- U.S. Equal Employment Opportunity Commission

  (800) 669–4000
  www.youth.eeoc.gov

For information about benefits for injured workers:

- North Carolina Industrial Commission

  (800) 688-8349
  www.ic.nc.gov

The information in this factsheet reflects your State and/or Federal labor laws as of 2010, whichever are more protective. The more protective laws usually apply. For current information, check with your state agencies listed in this handout.

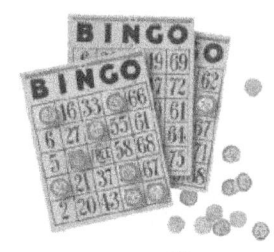

Labor Law Bingo: Board #1

8 hours	7 PM	18 years old	Box crusher	18 hours
The employer	Medical treatment	North Dakota Wage and Hour Division	North Dakota Human Rights Division	3 hours
53,000 teens	$_____ an hour	FREE SPACE	Safe and healthy workplace	Driving a vehicle
16 years old	Work permit	Load/unload trucks	9 PM	Follow safety rules
No	8 hours	Cleaning products	Yes	7 AM

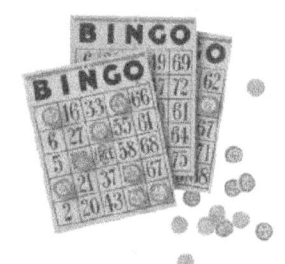

Labor Law Bingo: Board #2

Follow safety rules	8 hours	Whenever you start a new job	$_____ an hour	Protective equipment
8 hours	The employer	18 hours	North Dakota Human Rights Division	Medical treatment
7 PM	Cook	FREE SPACE	Fork Lift	OSHA
18 years old	Discarded needles	7 AM	9 PM	3 hours
North Dakota Wage and Hour Division	16 years old	Roofing	Work permit	Yes

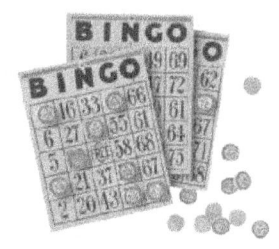

Labor Law Bingo: Board #3

	Lost wages $	18 years old	Handle, serve, or sell alcohol	3 hours
Follow safety rules				
North Dakota Wage and Hour Division	Load/unload trucks	7 AM	7 PM	16 years old
No	Yes	FREE SPACE	OSHA	8 hours
$_____ an hour	Box crusher	8 hours	9 PM	Cleaning products
18 hours	Protective equipment	Work permit	The employer	North Dakota Human Rights Division

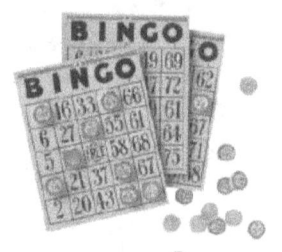

Labor Law Bingo: Board #4

8 hours	16 years old	The employer	Work permit	No
18 hours	$_____ an hour	Discarded needles	Follow safety rules	Box crusher
Yes	Driving a vehicle	FREE SPACE	9 PM	North Dakota Human Rights Division
Load/unload trucks	Lost wages $	53,000 teens	Whenever you start a new job	8 hours
7 PM	Protective equipment	North Dakota Human Rights Division	18 years old	3 hours

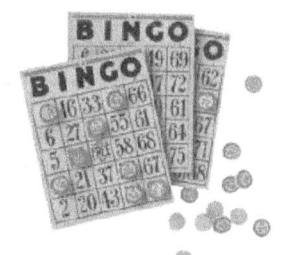

Labor Law Bingo: Board #5

		18 years old		18 hours
OSHA	No	(cake)	(moon) 9 PM	(clock)
The employer	North Dakota Wage and Hour Division	North Dakota Human Rights Division	$_____$ an hour	16 years old (cake)
(pot) Cook	Yes	FREE SPACE	53,000 teens	Whenever you start a new job
8 hours (clock)	Protective equipment	(moon) 7 PM	(forklift) Fork Lift	3 hours (clock)
(sun) 7 AM	Follow safety rules	(hand with cleaning spray) Cleaning products	(roof) Roofing	8 hours (clock)

Labor Law Bingo: *Board #6*

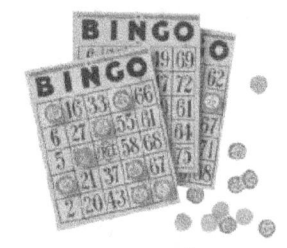

3 hours	Safe and healthy workplace	Protective equipment	North Dakota Human Rights Division	18 hours
North Dakota Wage and Hour Division	18 years old	Medical treatment	$_____ an hour	16 years old
Cook	Yes	FREE SPACE	8 hours	Work permit
Driving a vehicle	Whenever you start a new job	7 PM	OSHA	Report unsafe conditions
7 AM	Meat slicer	53,000 teens	The employer	8 hours

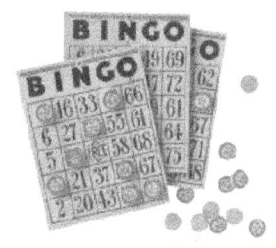

Labor Law Bingo: Board #7

Follow safety rules	Load/unload trucks	Whenever you start a new job	Handle, serve, or sell alcohol	18 hours
8 hours	Cleaning products	7 AM	Fork Lift	16 years old
Work permit	No	FREE SPACE	North Dakota Wage and Hour Division	8 hours
$_____ an hour	North Dakota Human Rights Division	The employer	Medical treatment	18 years old
Protective equipment	Yes	3 hours	7 PM	OSHA

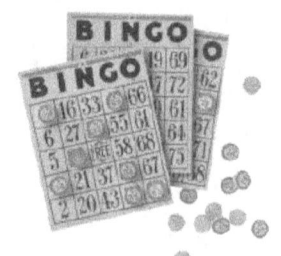

Labor Law Bingo: Board #8

Follow safety rules	8 hours	18 years old	Box crusher	18 hours
Medical treatment	Handle, serve, or sell alcohol	9 PM	Discarded needles	Work permit
3 hours	53,000 teens	FREE SPACE	OSHA	Load/unload trucks
$_____ an hour	16 years old	North Dakota Human Rights Division	7 AM	7 PM
The employer	No	Yes	8 hours	North Dakota Wage and Hour Division

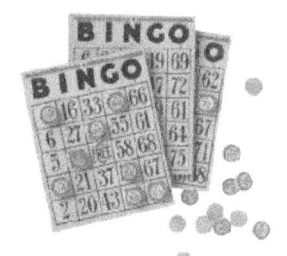

Labor Law Bingo: Board #9

OSHA	Yes	9 PM	Meat slicer	18 hours
16 years old	Work in manufacturing	3 hours	North Dakota Wage and Hour Division	North Dakota Human Rights Division
7 AM	Work permit	FREE SPACE	Safe and healthy workplace	53,000 teens
7 PM	8 hours	Cleaning products	8 hours	$_____ an hour
Driving a vehicle	18 years old	Follow safety rules	The employer	Lost wages $

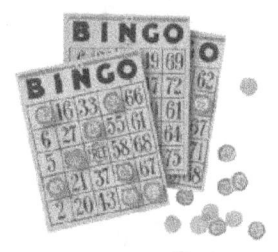

Labor Law Bingo: Board #10

		18 years old	North Dakota Human Rights Division	18 hours
The employer	Roofing			
Lost wages $	Discarded needles	7 AM	No	Load/unload trucks
3 hours	Box crusher	FREE SPACE	OSHA	9 PM
$_____ an hour	53,000 teens	16 years old	8 hours	7 PM
8 hours	Report unsafe conditions	Yes	Safe and healthy workplace	North Dakota Wage and Hour Division

Labor Law Bingo: Board #11

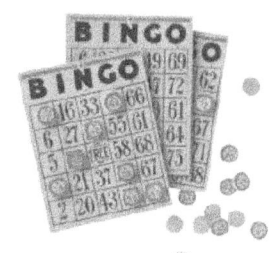

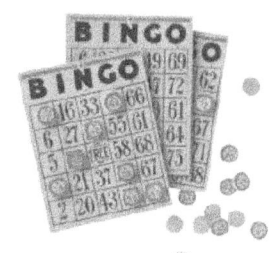 7 AM	18 hours	OSHA	Cleaning products	$_____ an hour
16 years old	Protective equipment	North Dakota Human Rights Division	18 years old	3 hours
8 hours	Load/unload trucks	FREE SPACE	Whenever you start a new job	Yes
Follow safety rules	Work permit	Driving a vehicle	7 PM	The employer
53,000 teens	No	Meat slicer	8 hours	9 PM

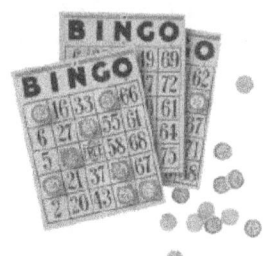

Labor Law Bingo: Board #12

Work permit	Load/unload trucks	18 hours	7 PM	The employer
7 AM	16 years old	North Dakota Wage and Hour Division	Yes	$_____ an hour
Meat slicer	Follow safety rules	FREE SPACE	Discarded needles	8 hours
8 hours	No	18 years old	Protective equipment	Roofing
9 PM	3 hours	OSHA	Lost wages $	Whenever you start a new job

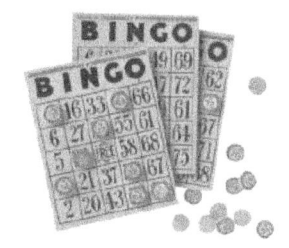

Labor Law Bingo: Board #13

3 hours	8 hours	18 years old	Handle, serve, or sell alcohol	OSHA
The employer	18 hours	7 AM	Cleaning products	16 years old
Work permit	Yes	FREE SPACE	North Dakota Human Rights Division	Meat slicer
$_____ an hour	Lost wages $	7 PM	8 hours	Follow safety rules
Whenever you start a new job	No	Load/unload trucks	9 PM	Protective equipment

Elena's Story

Scene: Sandwich shop. Elena is a 15-year-old high school student. Mr. Johnson is her supervisor, and Joe is one of her co-workers. It is Thursday evening.

Mr. Johnson: Elena, Andre just called in sick so I need you to work extra hours. I'd like you to stay until 10 tonight.

Elena: But Mr. Johnson, I have a test tomorrow and I need to get home to study.

Mr. Johnson: I'm really sorry, but this is an emergency. If you want to work here you have to be willing to pitch in when we need you.

Elena: But I've never done Andre's job before.

Mr. Johnson: Here's what I want you to do. First, go behind the counter and take sandwich orders for a while. Ask Joe to show you how to use the meat slicer. Then, when it gets quiet, go mop the floor in the supply closet. Some of the cleaning supplies have spilled and it's a real mess.

Later: Elena gets the mop and goes to the supply closet.

Elena: Hey, Joe! Do you know what this stuff spilled on the floor is?

Joe: No idea. Just be careful not to get it on your hands. You really should wear gloves if you can find any. Andre got a rash from that stuff last week.

Developing Your Role Play

1. Discuss with the class what laws are being violated here.

2. Work in your small group to come up with a different ending to the story. Choose one problem in the story to focus on. Think about these three questions:

   • How should Elena approach her supervisor about these problems?

   • What are the different ways her supervisor might respond?

   • Where else could Elena get help?

3. Practice role playing your ending with your group. You will perform for the class later.

Evaluation

Please answer these questions to help us evaluate how much you have learned.
You don't need to give your name.

1. The law says your employer must give you training about health and safety hazards on your job and how to prevent them.

    ☐ True   ☐ False   ☐ Don't know

2. The law sets limits on how late you may work on a school night if you are under 16.

    ☐ True   ☐ False   ☐ Don't know

3. If you are 16 years old, you are allowed to drive a car on public streets as part of your job.

    ☐ True   ☐ False   ☐ Don't know

4. If you're injured on the job, your employer must pay for medical care.

    ☐ True   ☐ False   ☐ Don't know

5. How many teens get seriously injured on the job in the U.S.?

    ☐ One per day   ☐ One per hour   ☐ One every 10 minutes   ☐ Don't know

6. If you had a health and safety problem on the job, what are two things you'd do?

    _____

    _____

7. Name at least two new things you learned about health and safety:

_____

_____

8. What did you like best about this health and safety training?

_____

_____

9. What suggestions do you have for improving this health and safety training?

_____

_____

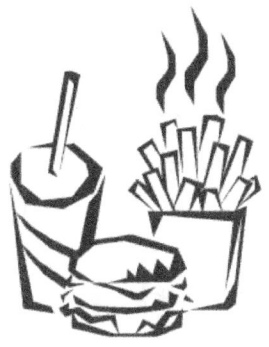

Hazards in the Fast Food Restaurant

HAZARD	EFFECT	POSSIBLE SOLUTIONS
Safety Hazards		
Cooking equipment	Burns or electric shocks	• Keep appliances in safe condition • Have guards around hot surfaces • Wear gloves or mitts
Hot grease	Burns	• Use grease pans that dump automatically • Have splash guards • Wear protective clothing
Slicers and powered cutting equipment	Cuts	• Must be 18 or older to use • Keep guards in place • Get proper training • Turn off when cleaning
Slippery floors	Slips or falls	• Clean up spills quickly • Use floor mats
Chemical Hazards		
Dishwashing products	Skin contact may cause irritation or dermatitis	• Use safer products • Wear gloves
Cleaning products	Some vapors cause headaches and other health problems; skin contact may cause irritation or dermatitis	• Use safer products • Wear gloves when necessary • Have good ventilation
Other Health Hazards		
Contact with public	Stress; criminal violence; robbery	• Have adequate security • Schedule at least two people per shift • Use barriers where money is handled • Get customer service training
Standing for long periods	Back injuries; varicose veins	• Use floor mats • Take regular breaks • Rotate jobs
Bending, reaching, stretching, and lifting	Muscle strains or sprains	• Keep heavy items on lower shelves • Rotate jobs • Use helpers

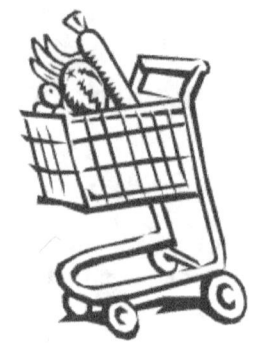

Hazards in the Grocery Store

HAZARD	EFFECT	POSSIBLE SOLUTIONS
Safety Hazards		
Box cutters	Cuts	• Cut properly • Store properly
Box crushers	Various body injuries	• Must be over 18 to use • Get proper training
Sharp knives	Cuts	• Keep in good condition • Cut properly • Store Properly
Deli slicers	Cuts	• Must be 18 or older to use • Keep guards in place • Get proper training • Turn off when cleaning
Chemical Hazards		
Cleaning products	Some vapors cause headaches and other health problems; skin contact may cause irritation or dermatitis	• Use safer products • Wear gloves when necessary • Have good ventilation
Other Health Hazards		
Checkout scanners	Muscle, tendon, or nerve injuries	• Redesign checkstands • Take regular breaks • Rotate jobs
Bending, reaching, stretching, and lifting	Muscle strains or sprains	• Use machinery instead • Keep heavy items on lower shelves • Get proper training • Rotate jobs • Use helpers
Cold temperatures (in cold storage areas, freezers)	Frostbite	• Limit time working in cold areas

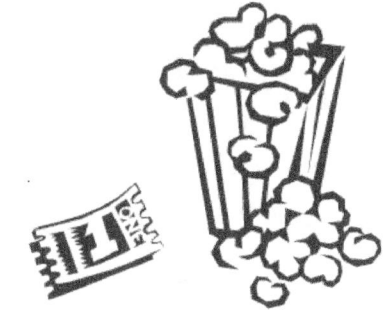

Hazards in the Movie Theater

HAZARD	EFFECT	POSSIBLE SOLUTIONS
Safety Hazards		
Popcorn, hot dog, and coffee machines	Burns or electric shocks	• Keep appliances in safe condition • Wear gloves or mitts
Slippery floors	Slips or falls	• Clean up spills quickly • Use floor mats
Ladders	Falls	• Must be 16 or older to use • Use safe ladders • Get proper training
Chemical Hazards		
Cleaning products	Some vapors cause headaches and other health problems; skin contact may cause irritation or dermatitis	• Use safer products • Wear gloves when necessary • Have good ventilation
Other Health Hazards		
Contact with public	Stress; criminal violence; robbery	• Have adequate security • Schedule at least two people per shift • Use barriers where money is handled • Get customer service training • Rotate jobs
Dark environments	Eyestrain; slips or falls	• Use flashlights
Standing for long periods	Back injuries; varicose veins	• Use floor mats • Take regular breaks • Rotate jobs

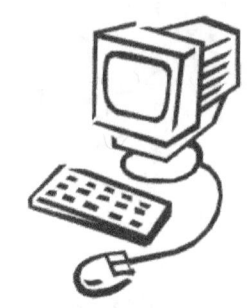

Hazards in the Office

HAZARD	EFFECT	POSSIBLE SOLUTIONS
Safety Hazards		
Cords and loose carpeting areas	Tripp ing	• Don't run cords through public • Keep carpets secured
Unsecured furniture	Can fall in earthquake	• Secure bookcases, file cabinets etc.
Overloaded electric circuits	Fire	• Have enough outlets
Chemical Hazards		
Ozone from copiers	Breathing difficulty; headaches; dizziness	• Place copiers in separate area • Have good ventilation
Poor indoor air quality	Breathing difficulty; headaches; dizziness	• Have good ventilation
Other Health Hazards		
Computer keyboards and mice	Tendon and nerve problems	• Use adjustable chairs and workstations • Have good posture • Take regular breaks
Computer monitors	Eyestrain	• Position monitor correctly • Adjust monitor properly • Take regular breaks
Sitting for long periods of time	Back pain	• Use proper chairs • Have good posture • Take regular breaks
Repetitive, boring work	Stress	• Rotate jobs

National Institute for Occupational Safety and Health

Centers for Disease Control and Prevention

recognizes . . .

for successfully completing the basic skills training course in
workplace safety and health

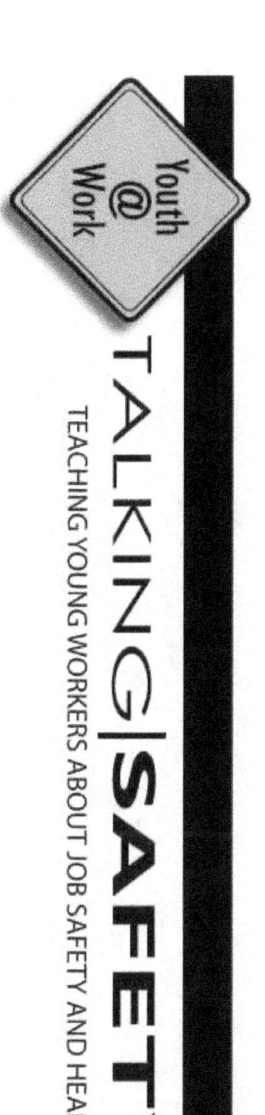

TALKING|SAFETY

TEACHING YOUNG WORKERS ABOUT JOB SAFETY AND HEALTH

www.cdc.gov/niosh/topics/youth

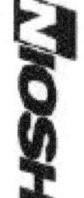

YOUNG WORKER SAFETY RESOURCE CENTER
www.youngworkers.org

Instructor

Date

www.ingramcontent.com/pod-product-compliance
Lightning Source LLC
Chambersburg PA
CBHW080413290526
45791CB00008BA/2251